Handling Death and
Bereavement at Wo

David Charles-Edwards

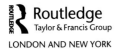

Routledge
Taylor & Francis Group

LONDON AND NEW YORK

A first edition of this book was published as Bereavement at Work
in 2000 by Gerald Duckworth & Co. Ltd.
First published 2005 by Routledge
2 Park Square, Milton Park, Abingdon, Oxon OX14 4RN
Tel: +44 020 7017 6000
Fax: +44 020 7017 6699

Simultaneously published in the USA and Canada
by Routledge
270 Madison Ave, New York, NY 10016

Routledge is an imprint of the Taylor & Francis Group

© 2005 David Charles-Edwards

Typeset in Baskerville by
Keystroke, Jacaranda Lodge, Wolverhampton
Printed and bound in Great Britain by
TJ International, Padstow, Cornwall

British Library Cataloguing in Publication Data
A catalogue record for this book is available from the British Library

Library of Congress Cataloging in Publication Data
A catalog record for this book has been requested

ISBN 0-415-34724-6 (hbk)
ISBN 0-415-34725-4 (pbk)

Handling Death and Bereavement at Work

An estimated 3,500 people die every day in the UK. Individuals' deaths may affect the workplace in many ways. If an employee dies or a partner of an employee, managers and colleagues will need to deal sensitively with the difficult issues that arise from death. How should one refer to what has happened? What influence does religion have? How much time for emotional recovery is reasonable? These are just some of the challenging questions that are addressed in this book, and other pertinent issues are discussed, including what to do in the event of a sudden death at work, managing staff with terminal illness, and practical tasks after death.

Handling Death and Bereavement at Work breaks new ground in placing bereavement on the management agenda rather than leaving a company's response to chance. This revised edition is an essential guide for anyone in an organisation who has to take responsibility in the event of death: managers, human resource and occupational health specialists, welfare officers and trade union representatives. It is also valuable reading for bereavement support workers and counsellors.

David Charles-Edwards is an experienced management consultant and counsellor in the field of leadership, relationships, diversity, change and loss. A former Industrial Society adviser, he has also led the personnel function in two health authorities and managed the British Association for Counselling (now BACP).

'This tremendously readable book contains a wealth of helpful and practical insights described simply and with great dignity and sensitivity.'

Chris Underhill MBE, Director, BasicNeeds

'I have personally lived with the guilt of failing to discuss the realities of death with my employer and workplace colleagues, and I now realise it was foolhardy not to share my pent up emotions.

This book has taken death and bereavement from the darkness into the light, and it will help shop stewards as well as managers and others ensure that the right kind of support is offered to people at work who are bereaved or struggling with a terminal illness. As one former General Secretary of my union said, trade unionists must look after their members from the cradle to the grave.'

Sir Bill Morris, General Secretary,
Transport and General Workers Union 1991–2003

'A source of ideas, insight and information which is likely to sustain managers, human resource specialists, staff representatives and colleagues as well as the bereaved over a long period of time.'

Peter Twist, former Chief Superintendent, Metropolitan Police

'Cogent and detailed descriptions of the underlying patterns associated with bereavement at work are dealt with in an accessible language and contain vivid accounts of real life experiences.'

Ross Warburton, Warburtons Limited

'Line managers and HR managers alike will be well advised to invest the time that it takes to read this carefully and sensitively written book, which explores a subject that is still too often shrouded in taboo and ignored in the workplace, and to act on the sound advice that it contains.'

Simon Armson, psychotherapist and former chief executive, The Samaritans

'An incredible amount of invaluable, practical and inspirational material is contained in these pages of sensitive and authoritative text . . . this guide cannot be too highly recommended for its practical comprehensive content and sincere, considerate approach.'

Occupational Health & Safety

'The anatomy of grief is dealt with especially well . . . a most humane, practical and good value for money publication.'

Health & Safety At Work

'For HR/personnel managers it will be an invaluable reference; for bereavement support workers it will provide added insight into the complex web of pressures a bereaved person may experience in what they often call the 'real' world of their work. This book, very helpfully, locates bereavement well and truly in that real world.'

Bereavement Care

IN MEMORY OF
HER BELOVED HUSBAND
DONALD WHYTE
DROWNED AT PORT ELLEN LIGHTHOUSE
1ST JANY 1916 AGED 53
ALSO THEIR SONS DANIEL WHYTE
DROWNED AT PORT ELLEN LIGHTHOUSE
1ST JANY 1916 AGED 17
PRIVATE DUGALD WHYTE 10TH A.& S.H.
KILLED IN ACTION 16TH DECR 1915 AGED 21
INTERRED IN MAPLE COPSE CEMETERY
ZILLEBEKE, NEAR YPRES, BELGIUM
LANCE CPL WALTER WHYTE 2ND A.& S.H.
KILLED IN ACTION 18TH AUGT 1916 AGED 20
INTERRED IN HIGH WOOD, NEAR MONTAUBAN, FRANCE
JOHN, WHO DIED IN INFANCY.
AND ROBERT
DIED 17TH JUNE 1933, AGED 28 YEARS
BETSY FERGUSON
DIED 8TH MAY 1935, AGED 69 YEARS
WIFE OF THE ABOVE DONALD WHYTE
THEIR DAUGHTER JESSIE
DIED 15TH AUGT 1950, AGED 52 YEARS

From a gravestone, Port Ellen, Islay in the Scottish Inner Hebrides.
© Keith Cocker. Image reproduced with kind permission of Keith Cocker.

Contents

About the author

David Charles-Edwards is a management consultant specialising in leadership, diversity, relationship and team building and counselling skills at work and is an associate of Trans4mation. He is married to Alison Parry and they have two sons, Owen and Samuel. He is also father of Anna, his daughter from his first marriage to Janet Hallpike, who died in 1966.

David formerly managed the British Association for Counselling (now the British Association for Counselling and Psychotherapy), before which he headed the NHS personnel functions, first in Hackney in London and then in Oxfordshire. His earlier work experience included being an adviser with The Industrial Society (now The Work Foundation), marketing research with the Metal Box Company, being a curate in Putney, south London, national service in the Royal Artillery, being a Prison Officer at HMP, Pentonville and shop officeman in the British Railways Iron Foundry in Crewe. David also jointly edited the 1st edition of *The Handbook of Counselling in Britain* with Windy Dryden and Ray Woolfe (Routledge, 1989).

His counselling experience includes training in re-evaluation counselling and in relationship counselling with Relate. He is an ordained minister in the Church of England.

Trans4mation is a management consultancy concerned with organisational and individual workplace training and development. (P.O. Box 44, Evesham, WR11 4ZJ, UK; www.trans4mation.com; david.charles@trans4mation.com).

Acknowledgements

This book has come out of my work with many clients, both individual and corporate, as well as my own experience and reading. I want to acknowledge them and also especially Alison, my wife, a hospice nurse and author of *The Nursing Care of the Dying Patient*, Peter Twist, formerly of the Metropolitan Police, and Peter McKenzie for their supportive and challenging help. I am especially grateful to John Flouch in his encouragement to write the 1st edition of this book, which was published by CEPEC, the management consultancy that he founded and with whom I was an associate consultant at the time. This book is built on that. I am also grateful to Karen Bowler, Cathy Hambly and others at Routledge for friendly, constructive and tolerant collaboration.

Since the first edition, Lucy Wetton has completed a study into *The Individual and Organisational Responses to Coping with Bereavement in the Workplace* as her final year dissertation for her BA Honours in Human Resource Management, published by the Southampton Institute in May 2003. I am grateful for her permission to draw on and at times quote from this and am pleased that her conclusions were in line with the thrust of this book.

The case studies and mini case studies in this book are drawn from the experience of real people but fictionalised in name and some of the detail to maintain confidentiality. The exception to this is where people have contributed and agreed to their real names being used, which applies where a surname is used.

Thanks also to Dr. Robert Abbott, Derek Avery, Tim Barton, Simon Burne, Ashley Callaghan, Debbie Collins, Maureen Hanson, Tam Kearney, Annie Kiff-Wood of Cruse Bereavement Care, Annie and Titus Mercer, Sue and Tony Pasternak, Tim Pears, Graham Powell, Judyann Roblee, Wendy Robinson, Hugh Scurfield, Anna Thomas, Jane Trinder, Chris Underhill and Kay Walker for the various ways they have influenced what I think and feel about this subject. In some cases they have contributed directly.

I am also grateful to Keith Cocker, whose photograph of a gravestone in Port Ellen on the Hebridean Island of Islay illustrates vividly the heartrending toll that dangerous work can taken of particular families and communities.

Colin Parry of the Warrington Project, Simon Armson and Norman Keir of the Samaritans were also greatly supportive in different ways.

None of these people, however, can share with me the responsibility for this book's deficiencies.

This book is not written for counsellors, but it does draw on my counselling experience and is about the use of counselling skills by all kinds of people in their work. The book draws on and is limited by my life experience, which includes that of managing and being managed as well as my counselling training and work. My counselling approach is predominantly person-centred, although I have also received training with a strong psychodynamic basis and am influenced by other approaches, which I respect, including Transactional Analysis (TA). I also draw on my experience as a client, counsellor and trainer in re-evaluation counselling.

A reviewer of the 1st edition of this book was concerned that it was too coloured by the fact of my being a priest and that I introduced the 'transpersonal' factor in the way I treat the subject. While discussing this issue further in Chapter 12, let me say here that the book is written from the perspective of diversity and empathy, and I hope that comes through. For many people the spiritual, religious and transpersonal are all meaningless concepts and resonate neither in their experience nor their outlook. For many others, this is not the case. To empathise means, being prepared and able to communicate respect, verbally and non-verbally, and hopefully understanding of people, irrespective of whether what they do or do not believe chimes with our own standpoint. It follows that it would defeat the empathic purpose of a book such as this to proselytise from a particular religious or non-religious perspective.

Reference

Charles-Edward, A. (1983) *The Nursing Care of the Dying Patient*, Beaconsfield, Beaconsfield Publishers.

Foreword

Ross Warburton,
Warburtons Limited

Ten years ago, after the New Year break, I returned to work to discover that a close colleague's son had been killed in a road accident in the early hours of New Year's Day morning. He'd had a row with his father, picked up the car keys and driven off, never to return. The sense of personal devastation was colossal, almost too big to look square in the eye. As his boss and a member of the family who owned the business, I felt an enormous sense of duty and sympathy towards him, but a great lack of personal skills to express these adequately. I am not alone, I fear. Many managers and leaders of businesses are great at the hard skills of managing performance and do their level best when it comes to coping with the special challenges posed when colleagues at work suffer personal difficulty. In the case of death, though, we are often found to be wanting at the time we are most needed.

David Charles-Edwards' book provides a crutch for all of us, who want to help but don't know the 'right' way to do it. His cogent and detailed descriptions of the underlying patterns associated with bereavement at work are dealt with in an accessible language and contain vivid accounts of real-life experiences. It is a practical guide for what has for too long been a taboo subject.

Introduction

Peter Twist, former Chief Superintendent, Metropolitan Police Service

Dealing with death or bereavement is one of life's greatest challenges. Yet we can so easily feel singularly ill-prepared for it. Death impacts on the workplace in many ways and this book breaks new ground in placing it on the management agenda.

In our role as manager, human resource specialist, trades union or staff association representative or colleague, we might cause great hurt or offence if we get it wrong. The eyes and ears of shocked and distressed people may be on us, especially if we occupy a position of leadership or influence. On the other hand, if we handle the issue well, we are helping people at their most vulnerable and demonstrating that we mean it when we talk the talk of being concerned for other people at work, as well as the organisation's success, however that might be measured. Sadly, it is often only when it happens to us that the learning begins: the feeling of being unsure of what to do or say may be matched only by the helplessness felt by the colleague concerned.

I hope that this book will be available from human resource, occupational health and welfare staff to others, especially line managers, senior staff and trades union and staff representatives. It is not necessary to read the whole book at first but use its contents pages to help with most immediate needs and concerns.

I was keen to support its development after working with David Charles-Edwards, who has supported, trained, coached and counselled people for over 25 years. I attended a workshop led by David and his wife, Alison, shortly after the death of my father. Knowing that one of my police officers at work was terminally ill, I sensed that a book based on the fruits of their experience might be timely for many people who want to be helpful but are struggling to know how to be so in the workplace.

Some readers may find swings from reflecting on the nature of death and bereavement to practical issues a little disconcerting, but such is the nature of death and bereavement. Anyone in a position of responsibility at work may find himself or herself becoming immersed in the details of informing others of a death and making arrangements for a funeral. What follows is a journey of many months or years of helping colleagues, as well as oneself, to come to terms with it. For this reason this book, while it can be read from the beginning to the end, is also of use as a reference and workbook, and a unique blend of information, ideas and insight. But before the book starts in some detail, you may find the contents pages helpful to guide you to where to start reading, which may not necessarily be from the beginning, depending on the situation you are dealing with.

The checklists that follow in Section 6 at the end of the book may also be a useful starting point for some readers. David has designed them to be copied and handed to colleagues according to their needs; an idea that deserves the usual acknowledgement to this book and its publisher.

Long after we have retired, or died, colleagues are more likely to remember us for the tact and sympathy we exercised in relation to bereavement at work than for anything else we did. Similarly, if we cause hurt or offence, people may never forget it. I commend this book to all who are determined to make even the most challenging moments in our working lives a positive experience.

For Samuel, Owen, Rosa and Maya and the future

And in loving memory of two remarkable women, who died before their time,

Janet Charles-Edwards, née Hallpike, 1939–1966
and
Melinda Cassel Powell, 1953–1999

Dealing with loss and bereavement

Chapter 1

What are loss and bereavement?

- 'Nobody dies wishing that they had spent more time at the office'
- Defining bereavement
- The task of bereavement
- Multiple losses
- Secondary losses, at and away from work
- The impact of bereavement on relationships
- 'In mourning'
- Collective grieving – public and private
- Dismissal as loss

'NOBODY DIES WISHING THAT THEY SPENT MORE TIME AT THE OFFICE'

In informal discussion at a recent leadership development workshop, the work–life balance issue came up among a bunch of managers. They all felt that it was a struggle to have a reasonable life outside work and still demonstrate credibly the commitment and passion for their business that was expected of them. It's a common disease in organisations and a dilemma for the people who work in them. Equally, 'nobody dies wishing that they spent more time at the office' is a thought that many people have, even if it sometimes feels too heretical to speak out loud in a workaholic culture. Death pushes us to sort out and re-evaluate what is really important: that is one of its gifts, even if for some it comes too late to do much with the new insights that can emerge from a brush with death, our own or someone else's.

Bereavement provides us with at least a small opportunity to show our human commitment to other people, irrespective of status, at work. But beyond all of that, there is a deep sense in which we are all equal as human beings. You do not have to be religious to be moved by the sentence from the funeral service: *We brought nothing into this world, and we take nothing out.*[1] Bereavement provides us not only with an opportunity but also a responsibility to support those affected by death for their sakes and that of the motivational health of the organisation.

DEFINING BEREAVEMENT

Bereavement has been described as the process of adapting to loss incurred through death.[2] It involves grief, which can feel overwhelming in the case of someone important to you. Grief itself varies, according to a number of factors, such as the depth of the relationship and how timely the death may or may not have been. The dictionary[3] equates being bereaved with being bereft, which means to take away, especially by death. Bereavement can also mean that we have lost something or someone. So it can feel either active or passive or both. We look further at efforts to make sense of this in Chapters 5 and 11. The active and passive meanings of death also mirror our active and passive responses considered in Chapter 2, Elements of Bereavement. Anger can stimulate a more active image of death as an enemy with whom we are drawn to struggle, while our sadness fits a more passive understanding of death about which we can do nothing.

Although bereavement usually refers to a loss through death, the word is sometimes applied to other kinds of loss. From childhood onwards we experience many kinds of loss, with which we have to cope, such as toys being broken, leaving home to go to school, a change of school, moving home or a parent leaving home through a relationship split. We experience the reaction of others to our distress, and also notice how they deal with their losses. Because the life expectancy of most pets is so much less than that of humans, virtually all of those who have pets experience their death. This early conditioning contributes to our emerging personality and helps to prepare the ground for the way that we learn to cope with losses, including, ultimately, our own mortality.

The actress Sheila Hancock has written, vividly about her relationship with her husband, John Thaw, about which she has said, "After John's death, I longed for a book that could honestly tell me how ghastly death is".[4] I hope that in this book the traps of pulling the punches and sentimentalising death have been avoided. On the other hand, our experience of dying and bereavement is integral to being alive with all the good that can bring. Grief is the price that we may pay for love, friendship and life itself.

THE TASK OF BEREAVEMENT

Bereavement is a journey, in and through which we need to come to terms with loss to the point where we can re-evaluate our life and move forward. This means beginning once more to value what we have, so that we become slowly a little less preoccupied with what has been lost. This is not to devalue the person who has died or what they meant to us, but is a matter of shifting the balance of attention towards what is still of value and makes our life worth living, even if at first this may be hard to find: there is hopefully still something to live for after all.

The idea of bereavement as a wound can also be helpful. A wound takes time to heal, and in the meantime it is important to avoid it becoming infected. We need to treat the wounded with great care. The subtle process of healing will, as with a physical wound, be happening to a considerable degree invisibly and unconsciously.

William Worden has described four tasks of mourning:[5]

Task 1: To accept the reality of the loss.
Task 2: To experience the pain or emotional aspects of the loss.
Task 3: To adjust to an environment in which the deceased is missing.
Task 4: To relocate the dead person within one's life and find ways to memorialise the person.

The latter is a response to the need to let go of the person, because there is also a deep sense that one will never, and indeed does not want to, forget a person who was important to us. Alice, aged 11, wrote down in her diary the day that her grandfather died: 'I will never forget Granddad'. And she didn't.

Some, perhaps many, past details about people are forgotten after they die, and this can be distressing, because it's as if it is only the memories of them that survive. We can forget just as much from the past about the living, but it matters less, because they are still there. Indeed, recalling old memories with friends can be a great pleasure as events are brought back that had been forgotten. Memory retention works differently for different people; it is not a measure of love or commitment to the person that has died.

The task of bereavement is to begin to withdraw emotional energy from the relationship with the person who has died and to reinvest it in existing and new relationships with the living. Before we can do that, a series of powerful responses needs to be worked through, allowing as much time as is needed, which is often rather longer than anticipated. During this process, the bereaved person may swing between grief, during which they are experiencing and coming to terms with their loss, and 'restoration', when they are focusing on the present and learning to cope with the future without the deceased.

Separating emotionally from a dead person is not easy, because the bonds we develop with each other are so powerful and necessary to our survival as social animals. We need the loyalty and commitment to each other, if our teams, work groups and families, as well as other working and personal relationships, are to function well. Arguably our passion for each other is a key to our success as a species. How many people bond with a sports team? Manchester United evokes a sense of 'we' and 'us', almost as powerful as any tribe, even among some who have been nowhere near the city. On a more personal level, this commitment in a family tends to be visible at the rituals surrounding birth, coming of age and marriage, as well as death. Many relatively trivial routines at home and at work can also strengthen our relationships with each other too. To break such powerful bonds of attachment, without denying the love that may outlast all the grieving until the survivor himself/herself dies, is a complex task.

A particularly poignant example of this is the death of a child, possibly in itself the hardest of all losses. When there are other siblings who survive, the parents have to grieve sufficiently but somehow maintain their eye on the ball of parenting and loving the children who survive. If they grieve inadequately, the surviving children may feel that they did not really care for their brother or sister, and perhaps by extension for them. If they grieve too wholeheartedly, they may feel that you have to die to be really loved. It is an extremely tough balance to strike.

For birds it seems much simpler, as the hedge sparrows feed the baby cuckoo, apparently oblivious of their own babies lying dead on the ground below, turfed out of the nest by the interloper. On the other hand, it is not necessarily only humans who mourn: elephants, for example, express what appears to be real grief at the death of one of their number.

During bereavement, this balancing and moving from grieving for the past into living in the present is necessary for survival, physical as well as emotional. Switching in and out of grief is often unpredictable to the bereaved person, let alone those who work or live with them, because it is usually an unconscious process, not easily managed to fit the convenience of external timetables, especially at first. A sign of the person moving through bereavement, however, is the sense that it is more controllable. The bereaved person becomes more able to choose when to move into grief and to be less at the mercy of being overcome suddenly and without warning in public or semi-public situations. To make this kind of progress usually means being able and prepared to allow the emotional pain to surface in order to speed up the healing process. Repressing pain does not make it go away, but rather tends to bury it deep, so that it grows like a destructive weed to take control and distort the way the mind works in the longer term.

MULTIPLE LOSSES

Multiple losses also complicate some bereavement. Recovering from a divorce, a redundancy or a death of someone close to us draws on the same pool of emotional and physical energy and resources. If two or even more such losses happen at the same time, they may feel overwhelming, whereas one of the losses on its own is likely to have been much more manageable. An attempt is made to quantify this in the 'Life Change Index',[6] at the end of Chapter 15. The Index illustrates the wide variety of loss, to which we are prone, by just living in a world, full of change, risk and danger. They can vary from the end of a relationship, job or career, to the break up of a family (due to emptying the nest, emigration or a feud), to the loss of a physical faculty or a limb through amputation or illness.

SECONDARY LOSSES, AT AND AWAY FROM WORK

Loss in bereavement may be further complicated by losses secondary to the primary loss of the person through death. If the deceased has been the major breadwinner, their surviving partner may experience the loss of the life-style they both enjoyed or the status that the other person made possible. If an only child dies, the man or woman is no longer a parent. A surviving parent finds that they may not feel so welcome at social occasions with former friends, insensitively dependent on socialising interminably in couples. The marginalising and even rejection of some bereaved people who have become single, by former apparently friendly couples, is the absolute opposite of genuine friendship. It is hurtful at a time when they are at their most vulnerable and is sadly far from rare.

A bereaved person may have to make various, sometimes quite profound, changes in the way they live and think about their lives, especially if the person was close in practical as well as in emotional ways. The life together has itself died with the loss of the other person. A new life has to be created without them. There follows, therefore, a period of adjustment and, quite possibly, learning or even training, which is interwoven with the process of grieving. Stroebe and Schut have depicted the tension in this 'dual process' in a helpful model:[7]

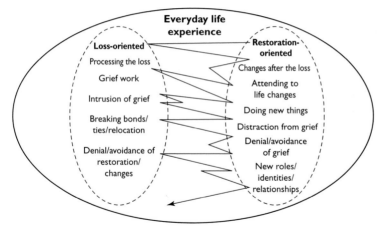

Figure 1 The dual process model of coping with bereavement
Source: Stroebe and Schut, 1999: 213

The bereavement process is seen as constantly moving from being preoccupied with the loss to putting that on one side for the moment and getting on with life, but there is a tension in shifting our energy between two such demanding sets of needs. If one predominates, it can lead, on the one hand, to repressing our grief and failing to allow it to begin to heal or, on the other hand, to neglecting the basis of our life for the future: work, health and key relationships.

This model is music to the ears of those who know that work is not for most people a luxury to be picked up when you feel like it. It is a necessity for the individual and society: work is necessary for survival. So the resolution-oriented tasks of the Stroebe and Schut model can be linked to the need to 'get on with things'. This is of course not just good for the organisation but can be therapeutic too for the bereaved person: a veritable win–win, so long as managers are aware that it is not the whole story of the longer-term working through a bereavement. On the other hand, some employees may lose their work, if only temporarily, as Annie Hargrave, quoted also in Chapter 3, did when she stopped her work as a counsellor because her 21-year-old son was diagnosed with an incurable form of cancer in July 2001. She subsequently wrote, 'It wasn't a difficult decision but it was a huge loss which came on top of this devastating blow to the core of my life. I lost my independent life, I lost the daily company of my colleagues, I lost the value of the involvement in the world of my vocation, I lost my income, which wasn't immediate, but was very significant. I lost the patients to whom I was very committed and I lost the experience of competence. I am competent and pleased to be so. Not perfect, but competent'.[8]

Such secondary losses may require resolute and enlightened compensatory changes in behaviour. New tasks may not fit gender stereotypes, which may have been part of the relationship previously. So the elderly person, with a minimal overlap of roles in their past relationship with the deceased person, learns to live alone and to master new skills: cooking, paying the bills, changing a plug, doing the shopping, using the lawn mower or washing machine. A young husband with a job that takes him away a lot may have to find new, possibly lower paid, work to be more available for the children and perhaps manage a tighter budget. A young mother may have to find work outside the home, possibly for the first time, without the children being neglected. She may even have to move to a smaller house in a different area if she cannot afford the mortgage. Children may have to change schools or no longer find anyone at home when they return from school.

> Sometimes neighbours can be wonderful. When I moved to Oxford to a new job with my nine-year-old daughter after my first wife's death, she usually came home from school two hours before I did. Although there were friends who came in from time to time, our retired next-door neighbour, Mrs. Bruce, always left some fresh sandwiches for her on the kitchen table, a signal that she could pop round if she had any worries. Looking back on those days, she has told me what a comfort that was, even though in reality she did not spend much time next door. Little things, coming with thoughtfulness and genuine concern, can mean a lot.

Even when we 'only' have to cope with a single death, we may through that death be experiencing a multitude of losses, such as companionship, support, a sexual relationship, co-parenting, help, knowledge, skills, shared interests, pleasure and laughter.

In the workplace, there may be a whole raft of secondary losses with the death of a colleague, including many, if not all, of the ones just mentioned. A secondary loss is thus one that comes as a by-product of the main loss.

Someone with whom we work closely dies and we find, for example, that we may have also lost:

- a fishing, drinking or bridge partner;
- someone who could sort out the computer when it goes wrong;
- someone else who could stand up to our boss, without him losing his temper;
- a person who knows what it is like to have worked for the company;
- a good sales person;
- a fellow fan of Bolton Wanderers;
- someone in the team with a sense of humour like mine;
- someone at work who got on with my wife and helped to make social occasions at work enjoyable for her.

THE IMPACT OF BEREAVEMENT ON RELATIONSHIPS

Fundamental to all good relationships is respecting and understanding each other – easy to write, but much less easy to do. This acceptance can, however, often feel particularly difficult in the face of bereavement.

Partnerships sometimes experience great pressure after bereavement due to the different ways each person responds. After the death of a close family member, one person may feel the need to talk and the other, with their own grief, may find it hard to listen. One partner may avoid the subject, for fear of upsetting the other, who in turn meanwhile longs to talk. One spouse may be more private and the other more public with their feelings. At the private end of the spectrum, the person may keep their grief to themselves, talking little to the other. The latter may want to talk and cry a lot with other people, rather than be on their own. One may greatly value unburdening with other people, whereas the other may want to keep it to themselves or to the two of them. One may seek some sexual comfort as consolation or even distraction, while the other may be repelled by any thought of sex at such a time.

This kind of difference can also find expression in planning the funeral arrangements. One person may want to personalise the funeral with favourite music, personal tributes and reminiscences, while the other may find more comfort in formality or a traditional format, in which the expression of grief can be minimised and thus kept as private as possible. People often seem to be drawn to someone temperamentally very different to themselves. The attraction of opposites consciously or unconsciously compensates for limitations in the individual. Looked at more positively, such synergy enhances the strength of what they have as a couple. When bereavement hits them, this does not make it easy for them to understand and meet each other's needs, particularly if both of them are exceptionally needy. Disappointment and even anger can build up, if it is not resolved through communication: at worst one person may feel disgust and contempt at the other's lack of restraint. 'It degrades the memory of our daughter.' On the other hand, the restraint of the other partner can be experienced as uncaring coldness. At such times of vulnerability, there can be a pull to believe that the other ought to be reacting in the same way and resentment that they are not doing so.

In all good relationships there needs to be a balance between support and encouragement, on the one hand, and challenging or confronting, on the other. Support provides the foundations on which mutual understanding and respect is built, so that challenges can be experienced as acceptable and hopefully constructive, rather than feeling like an antagonistic attack. This applies to relationships at work as much as it does in the family or in other parts of our life.

The following model graphically depicts the impact of bereavement on a partnership. Although it applies to partnerships, such as marriages and those between others with a long-term commitment to sharing their life with each other, it can also be related to strong working partnerships.

Stage 1: Two people come together to develop an interdependent rela-tionship. At an unconscious and a conscious level, people seem to be drawn to each other because of both their similarities and their differences. They may have striking physical facial similarities and shared values, beliefs or interests; but in personality and skills they may be very different. The result is that the partnership or team has a richness and strength that neither person had as individuals, even though their differences may be a source of conflict needing to be sorted out to an extent at this stage. In the field of work, there are numerous famous examples: Laurel and Hardy, Crick and Watson, Duke Ellington and Billy Strayhorn, Morecambe and Wise, and Redgrave and Pinsent. They had different partners in their private life, but they worked together so well because they complemented each other and became a team, a new unit. For this to work at its best, they moved towards:

Stage 2: They had got to know each other well enough and they had established a way of working or being with each other, so that they hardly had to think about it. Sometimes this understanding and knowledge were so powerful, they could predict each other's behaviour and thinking, so it almost becomes telepathic. The partners play to their strengths that can become exaggerated in the relationship. The opposite can also be true: each partner may become less confident, even deskilled in some areas, as they leave certain things to the other one. One of them dies and they are catapulted into:

Stage 3: They realise how they have come to depend on the other person and sometimes only feeling half-alive as a result themselves. At this point they may spasmodically look for an immediate replace-ment and prematurely try to recruit one, only to reject them because they never turn out to be the person they really want. They can be uncharacteristically promiscuous at this point, leading some others to feel bitter and rejected. One way or another, by going through the grieving process, they hopefully work towards:

Stage 4: They become something of a whole person again, though different from where they were on their life journey, when they were at Stage 1. At this point, they will be far readier (than in Stage 3) to move into a new relationship, in which there will be much less danger of their new partner forever being compared unfavourably with the perhaps idealised, deceased one. In the new relationship there will be different possibilities and differences too in how they complement each other.

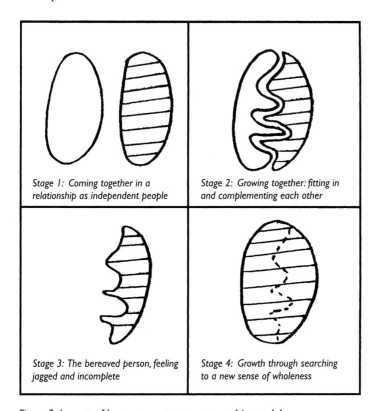

Stage 1: Coming together in a relationship as independent people

Stage 2: Growing together: fitting in and complementing each other

Stage 3: The bereaved person, feeling jagged and incomplete

Stage 4: Growth through searching to a new sense of wholeness

Figure 2 Impact of bereavement on a partnership model

Stephen and John had been together for nearly 10 years, and those who knew them thought of them as a great team, partly because they complemented each other so well. The sum was definitely greater than the parts! Within their relationship, however, those differences that were such a strength on good days were on bad days a source of conflict and tension, when they found it hard to accept each other.

Nevertheless, after John's death in a road traffic accident, Stephen found himself grieving as much for the creative spontaneity and even chaos as for the order in their relationship. The secondary losses he experienced included John's gift for fresh ideas, for reaching out to people and dealing assertively with the difficult ones. Without the reality of the day-to-day irritations in their relationship, he was able to see more clearly what a great team they were. He often asked himself why it should have taken John's death for him to get in touch with that realisation again.

'IN MOURNING'

Many people will experience bereavement without necessarily feeling the intensity of feelings described in this book. The words 'bereavement', 'grief' and 'mourning' are sometimes used almost interchangeably to describe our reaction to death. 'Grief' is a strong word for sorrow in the face of a major loss, whereas 'mourning' has two meanings: grieving itself or a period of time given over to grieving. The clothes worn to show grief when someone dies are an aspect of the latter, although that custom has diminished in the past generation or two.

On a personal basis, someone may be thought of as 'in mourning' for very variable periods: the time in which they are, or at least allow others to see that they are, preoccupied by their loss. Society also prescribes periods of mourning. In some cultures this may be a month, in others a few days. In England, for many, there is an unwritten convention that it lasts from the death to the funeral, after which the bereaved are expected to become more self-sufficient again and 'back to normal', as if they have used up their quota of sympathy. At its best, this norm gives permission to grieve openly and also a steer to move forward. The consequence of this subtle pressure is that people make great efforts to hide what may be reservoirs of grief from others as a social duty. It is as if a sign is required that they are strong enough to look after themselves and are free from the excesses of self-indulgence, which is the cruel veneer that is sometimes expected from what some think of as the bereaved, not least in the workplace that is more dysfunctional.

It is not a new phenomenon. In the Bible, the author of the Book of Isaiah [chapter 53, verse 3] writes of 'a man of sorrows, and acquainted with grief' or 'humbled by suffering', in the New English Bible translation.[9] It continues: 'and we hid as it were our faces from him; he was despised, and we esteemed him not'. In this we have an echo of the modern message to those who are in mourning that, if they want to be popular, they need to get over it fairly smartly. To praise a bereaved person for coping so well can sometimes deliver the same message. The subtext reads: coping well means not upsetting, depressing or embarrassing the rest of us by showing too much grief. Books such as this are hopefully reflecting as well as encouraging a change in our culture towards a more understanding and accepting attitude to those 'in mourning', so that they have to pretend less to those close to them at work or at home about how they are really feeling.

COLLECTIVE GRIEVING – PUBLIC AND PRIVATE

Bereavement is experienced individually and sometimes collectively. The isolation and loneliness felt can be particularly hard if you feel that nobody else cares deeply about the death of someone to whom you are very close. Nevertheless, in various ways and to various degrees grief can be shared: within a work team, a family or some other small or large circle of people. Its pain may have significance for us as a species, serving the function of binding the social group. Hence the importance of funerals for many people. We have a sense of what we value, and therefore need to look after with special care, partly though the intensity of our grief. So as a society we normally see the death of a child or young person as more tragic than that of an older person, especially if they have had their three score years and ten, or these days a score or more beyond that.

Public outpourings for the premature and violent deaths in the past century have been many: Gandhi, Steve Biko, President Kennedy and his brother Robert, Martin Luther King and even John Lennon. A dramatic example of collective grieving was the public response in Britain to the sudden death in a Paris car crash on 31 August 1997 of Diana, Princess of Wales. After a week of people queuing to get into my town centre church in Rugby to sign the Book of Remembrance and make donations to her charity, the service the following Sunday focused on her death. Several people were crying as they took their communion, and one young woman stayed behind, too upset to move. Asked if her tears were about Diana, she replied: 'They are partly but they are mainly for my father who died four months ago and I haven't realised how much I missed him till this week'. She explained further that it had struck her forcibly how it felt to her that, although she greatly loved her father, his death had not been properly acknowledged when it happened. In stark contrast, for Diana the crowds had gathered, reflected and spurred on by the media who selected her death to dominate their space. This outpouring of feelings brought home to many that if we really care about someone, they may also warrant, at least in their own circle of family and friends, the level of mourning that was focused towards Diana nationally and even internationally. For many her death felt a very personal loss, but for others there was a sense of her as a symbol of much that was good and beautiful, combined with the special tragedy of an avoidable and violent death to someone still young.

There was also a massive public response to each of the massacres in East Africa in Nairobi and Dar es Salaam or in Omagh, Northern Ireland in 1998, America in 2001, Bali in 2002 and Madrid in 2004. The bombs, which had killed and injured so many, united people in a strong sense of their common humanity.

These experiences parallel the way grief can totally preoccupy us as individuals, at least initially. In the case of terrorism, the anger that is part of the grief is often very near the surface. When death has been inflicted so cruelly, randomly and deliberately on so many by other human beings, there is an enormous desire for justice as well as fear of being a victim of the next random atrocity. War is bad enough but it is hopefully supported by some rationale such as that of the just war. There should also be a real attempt to stick to the Geneva Convention, treating prisoners humanely and minimising casualties, at least civilians, not that that gave much comfort to the inhabitants of Hiroshima, Nagasaki, Coventry and Dresden in the 1939–1945 war. It is ironic that modern warfare, conducted often by people who reject the savagery of medieval wars, ends up with greater civilian suffering. Inhumanity reaches new depths in genocide.

A public response to most atrocities is not only a way of sharing, albeit only in a relatively small way, the grief of the immediately bereaved. It is also a way for people to disassociate themselves from the atrocity so that the message is reinforced that only a tiny minority of unrepresentative monsters are engaged in such behaviour. The whole world has not gone mad. Such crumbs of comfort are not available to the victims of ethnic cleansing, where powerful majorities appear to turn on minorities, whether in Nazi Germany, Pol Pot's Cambodia, the Kurds, Rwanda, the Lords Resistance Army in northern Uganda, Kosova or East Timor.

British examples of traumas include those in 1989 in Sheffield at Hillsborough Stadium or two years earlier the sinking of the Herald of Free Enterprise. Colin and Wendy Parry have described movingly[10] the public response to the terrible murder of their son Tim and Johnathan Ball by the IRA bombing in Warrington, England on 20 March 1993.

When the media and members of the public, who did not know the people who have died, become involved in bereavement, it is as if they un-officially represent the community. At worst such attention can be intrusive and make the tragedy harder to bear; at best, for some, a real comfort that strangers apparently really cared about those who have died.

This role of representing the wider community can be fulfilled in a more discreet way by the work organisation, along with any other organisations associated with the person who has died, such as sporting, arts or other club or a voluntary, religious or political organisation. Ways in which the organisation can express such support are discussed in Chapter 13: 'How the organisation can help'.

At its root, bereavement is an intensely personal experience, even when it is shared. That sharing can be a mixture of shared grief and support from others, who are grieving less strongly themselves but who have a commit-ment to those mainly suffering the loss. The closer the bereaved person is to the one who has died, usually the more painful the loss is. It seems to be an unavoidable equation. The deeper the friendship or love we feel for each other, potentially the deeper is the pain and the longer the process of grieving is likely to be. But there is a paradox too: while on one level death changes everything in a relationship, on another level the experience of loss can often seem to change nothing of the feelings towards the person who has died. Edith Sitwell in some memorable lines wrote:

Love is not changed by Death
and nothing is lost
and all in the end is Harvest.[11]

The news that Emma had been killed the previous day in a car crash traumatised the whole working group in the open-plan office for a long time. She had been young, healthy and full of life. An empty desk, normally such a mundane phenomenon, became a focal point of disbelief and sadness. For a time it was left empty as her personal belongings were removed. Eventually, her successor was appointed to the uncomfortable task of stepping into 'dead woman's shoes', and making Emma's workspace her own.

Emma had been popular when alive, but her popularity became exaggerated in death, as the irritating aspects of her behaviour were mostly forgotten out of respect for her memory. After all, her colleagues were now free of those negative aspects; so, consequently, she became a harder act to follow than if she had lived and moved to another job.

In departmental gossip, her successor, Annabel, tended to be compared unfavourably with Emma, although a couple of people stuck up for her and went out of their way to make her feel welcome. They were the main ones to have quarrelled with Emma frequently and wanted to ensure that the guilt they felt after her death was not going to be repeated a second time. In any case they personally found Annabel a good deal easier to get along with.

Once Emma's death had been sufficiently mourned, her colleagues started to feel that they could accept Annabel as part of the team without feeling that they were betraying Emma. Had she not been killed but had taken off for a new life in another place, or got a better job, she would have been a much easier act to follow.

The way that such events are handled by management and colleagues can make a big difference to how the Annabels of this world work their way into a new job when they follow someone who has died or been killed.

DISMISSAL AS LOSS

When people are separated from their work for whatever reason, they are likely to experience something that may have much in common with bereavement. Of course some redundancies, for example, are much more traumatic than others, but so are some deaths. The emotional intensity felt varies a great deal. That depends on many circumstances, such as the behaviour of the company and the line manager, the support provided and available, as well as the external circumstances and aspirations of the staff involved.

A clue as to how enlightened employers are likely to behave in the face of death and bereavement may be their behaviour when they dismiss people through redundancy. Sometimes they can hardly wait to get people out of the building after informing them about their fate, having established that there are no alternative employment possibilities within the company. Until that moment the staff member may have been trusted, but once redundancy strikes they are regarded as potential saboteurs and thieves. So the chance of a decent departure and 'closure' is undermined.

'The beginning of motivating those who remain is influenced by how you treat those who go' is a slogan adopted in some of our managing change consultancy. It is a great mistake not to offer the latter time to process the ending of their job and farewells in the company. They usually need some opportunity, with reasonable support from colleagues and others, to collect their thoughts and feelings and begin to move towards the next chapter of their working lives. If effort has been made to build morale and team spirit in working groups, members of those groups cannot suddenly be expected to be indifferent to colleagues simply because they (or rather their jobs) are deemed surplus to requirements.

> Serious criminal allegations were made against Derek about events that had supposedly occurred 20 years before. Because the allegations, if proved, would have made him unsuitable for his present job in a charity, it was felt that he had to be suspended. However, his work performance had so far been exemplary. He was not in disgrace. Nothing had been proved. So the organisation maintained contact and found him some work to do from home. Later, after he had been cleared and was back at work, he said how cut off he had felt, as reciprocally had his colleagues.

With dismissal for misconduct, the norm would be to demand that the staff member depart at once because they have shown themselves to be unreliable and possibly dishonest. So guilt about them is often minimised because they have supposedly brought their fate upon themselves. Good managers, however, may feel some guilt or at least an element of personal responsibility in most dismissals on the grounds of misconduct or incompetence, because there has often been failure in such areas as selection, induction, training, motivation or supervision.

Work can be a sheet anchor, socially as well as financially, and a significant part of a person's identity, which is why losing it and a bereavement coming together can feel so catastrophic. 'It seemed like the end of the world.' It was the end of the previous world of meaning.

Notes

1 The 1st letter of Timothy, chapter 6, verse 7 in the New Testament of the Bible.
2 Worden, W. (1996) *Children and Grief*, New York and London: Guildford Press.
3 *New Generation Dictionary* (1981), London: Longman.
4 Hancock, S. (2004) *Two of Us: My Life with John Thaw*, London: Collins.
5 Worden, W. (1996), *ibid*.

6 *'Life Change Index' From Strategies in Self-Awareness*, London: The Marylebone Health Centre.

7 Stroebe, M. and Schut, H. (1999) 'The dual process model of coping with bereavement: rationale and description', *Death Studies*, vol 23, no. 3.

8 Hargrave, A. (2003) *Fit to Work*, Rugby: BACP in CPJ: Counselling and Psychotherapy Journal, 3: 2003.

9 *New English Bible* (1961) Oxford: Oxford University Press and Cambridge University Press.

10 Parry, C. and Parry, W. (1994) *Tim: An Ordinary Boy*, London: Hodder and Stoughton.

11 Whitaker, A. (ed.) (1984) *All in the End is Harvest: An Anthology for Those Who Grieve*, London: Darton, Longman and Todd in association with CRUSE.

Chapter 2

Aspects of bereavement

INTRODUCTION

The focus of this chapter is on the kind of grieving process that people tend to go through, although there is 'no road map for how executives (or anyone else) should deal with grief'.[1] Bereavement is such an individual experience that it is foolish to imagine we can describe with any precision the route that is to be taken beforehand. Colin Parry, for example, has written after the murder of his son, Tim, by the IRA in Warrington that he and his wife Wendy 'learned that people do not grieve according to schedules and timetables. There can be wild and irrational mood swings. There were times when grief and anger overcame me and she appeared calm and controlled. There were times when the raw emotion was hers, and I was numb and frozen'.[2]

In other circumstances, grief can strike like an arrow through the armour of coping at work or outside work. Sara Payne has described how, after the disappearance and subsequent discovery of the murdered body of her eight-year-old daughter Sarah, she was very different at home and in public.[3] Her public work included relating to the media, especially in the early days, in a way carefully calculated to recover Sarah unharmed if possible. She tried in her televised appeal to appear 'not raging or lamenting, or calling for the death penalty, but soothing and calm, trying to establish some kind of one-to-one relationship with the abductor, get across the idea that there was still a chance to step back from the darkness'. By her own account, her impressive strength in public contrasted with how she was at home. She lost the plot, alternating between over-protecting her children and neglecting the normal motherly roles. She let the house turn into a tip, often sitting in her dressing gown, chain-smoking, watching day-time television for hours. Along with the big issues, her book illustrates the sheer mess murder can make of daily life: dirty pots in the sink, stale milk in the fridge. 'It is messy, it is dark,' as Sara told the journalist Barbara Ellen. 'You spend your life going to places you don't want to go.'[4]

The more the experience of bereavement is understood, the more the feelings experienced can, however, be understood paradoxically as highly rational. They follow their own logic, even though they may seem unpredictable. Sara Payne had to get on with her life, initially with its total focus on the safe recovery of her daughter if humanly possible, requiring constant bursts of grit and adrenaline, but she also had to grieve – initially over the loss and then coming to terms with her daughter's terrible death. The toll that took on her energy would inevitably be massive. The washing up came nowhere against such priorities and relationships with the living can also seem secondary. As with so many couples, the toll on her relationship with her husband Michael was enormous. People who kill succeed in killing so much indirectly as well as directly.

The process is not easily switched off, like a gas fire, when people touched by death come to work, however hard they may try to control their feelings. If they were feeling 'fine' or overwhelmed yesterday, it does not mean that they will feel the same today. It can be like an emotional switchback, difficult to follow, especially in someone else, which is why it is so important to respect the person, however they are feeling, if you are trying to support them. That respect requires suspending judgement, but rather noticing and accepting how they are doing at any particular moment. In particular it is important not to try and imagine how you might be feeling in the same situation, because you do not know, you are not the same person and the situation is therefore not the same.

For some people, to be able to share what they are going through from time to time with others at work may be really helpful. At times this may even be necessary for them to feel that they can get through a working day. For others, their grieving may be more private or at least shared with family or friends away from the workplace.

RELIEF

Bereavement is not always completely unpleasant. The good memories that have been shared with the person who has died can make the experience sweet as well as bitter. Comfort can also be drawn from the way that other people express their love and admiration for the person who has died. In the words of one widow: 'I knew how much I loved him but I had no idea until he died how many people he worked with thought so much of him too'. The irony is that the deceased person may not have realised it either. Even allowing for an element of rose-tinted sentimentality, it sometimes takes someone's death for us to realise how much we valued them.

Relief can ameliorate the worst part of bereavement. The quality of life may have deteriorated to the point where death seemed to be the lesser of two evils or even the 'blessed relief' of stereotyped Victorian religion, devoted as it was so often to looking forward to a life after death. Alternatively, where the relationship was acrimonious, there may be a sense of liberation from conflict, quarrelling or nagging. Where the relationship felt claustrophobic, the freedom to choose to do what you want, rather than always being expected to fit into the incessant demands and preferences of a boss, colleague or partner, can be tremendous.

The relief can be very real even for what might seem trivial reasons. One widow, for example, told me after the death of her husband that she could choose what to watch on television and when to eat. It represented for her a basic independence that she enjoyed and had lost in her marriage. Relief does not, however, necessarily make the process easier. The relief can be complicated by guilt and by regret for what was missing from the relationship. The finality of death creates an inability to ever improve it. There can be an element of grieving for the unfulfilled hopes for the relationship that never was.

Most relationships, good as well as not so good, are characterised by ambivalence or mixed feelings towards each other. These are usually present at some level, even if unconscious, and are arguably healthy and necessary if the other person is a fallible, real human being. Additionally, people in relationships need space as well as closeness. At work, we may have had hopes and fantasies that a colleague or boss would be the perfect one, but getting to know them as real people involved the halo slipping. So there may be, at some level, a bit of relief amidst the grief.

DREAMS

As suggested in one of the checklists in section 6, bereaved people, even if they do not normally remember their dreams, may experience and perhaps recall particularly vivid dreams. The unconscious mind works on the feelings brought up by the loss, while asleep as well as awake and while the conscious part of the mind is at rest. When dreaming, the mind is freed from the constraints of logic to explore uninhibitedly feelings at their most intense. It can be sometimes helpful to just ask a person who is bereaved if they are dreaming differently since the death, because if they are, it can be reassuring to realise that it is not unusual. That does not protect them from the impact of the dreams, any more than friends and family can relieve people from waking grief, but simply from a possible added burden of thinking that they are abnormal.

While they are referred to elsewhere, some of the characteristics of dreams after bereavement and the themes that underpin them include the following:

■ Sometimes they seem to occur in that period between being asleep and awake.

- Sometimes the person who has died reappears in the dream as if they are still alive or have come back from the dead.
- Sometimes the person is there in the dream as if alive but the dreamer cannot communicate with them. Perhaps the person who has died cannot see or hear them or cannot be reached in some other way.
- Sometimes in the dream it is suggested that the person is still alive but living elsewhere with new family or friends.
- Sometimes the dreamer is searching for the person who has died, with or without eventual success.
- Sometimes very upsetting elements in the dying, from an accident or painful illness, are revisited and relived in the dream, sometimes repetitively.
- Sometimes the dream makes the dreamer feel guilty, and perhaps punished, for how they behaved towards the person who has died or for just still being alive.

THREE PHASES OF GRIEF

In the next section of this chapter on 'Ten elements of bereavement', grieving is described in more detail, but it may be helpful to simplify its essence. One example is to identify three main aspects:

Denial	■ shock, disbelief, fantasy and numbness, during which the significance or impact of the death may be minimised.
Emotional pain	■ experiencing grief through anger, depression, apathy, guilt, searching, pining and loneliness.
Acceptance	■ recovering interest in work and life, despite the loss of the deceased, and becoming ready to engage in new activities and relationships, relocating energy from the past into the future.

This movement from stage to stage and back again is characteristically an unconscious process. Consequently, the bereaved person does not usually feel as if they are in control of their mood changes, which can be so painful that we would be unlikely to choose consciously to enter them. So it can feel as if it is happening to us, outside our control, but it is a process necessary for recovering the possibility of happiness. Mood swings are a normal, perhaps barely noticed, part of human experience. What makes them remarkable in bereavement is their power. When the swing happens, it can feel like a setback. It is, however, just as likely to be a step forward, as conscious awareness of our feelings recurs and maybe some more of the pain from our loss is healed.

To describe the elements of bereavement can be both useful and also misleading. They can be put in an apparently logical sequence, but the reality is usually different. People move from one to another and then loop back to an earlier stage. Healing comes for many as the feelings come to the surface and begin to dissipate bit by bit. We may step backwards in order to deal with pain at a deeper level than before, now that we are ready for it. We may, however, also be propelled out of a stage, if only temporarily, because of the need for a break from its intensity and to get on with the rest of our life.

The ten emotional elements in the bereavement process described below can, therefore, be seen as some of the landmarks people may go past, though not necessarily in the order that they appear here. The order approximates to the route quite a few people discover that they follow, but it cannot be stated too strongly that the journey may vary. In summary, this may happen in any or all of the following four ways:

- The order may be different from that of the model.
- Going back to some elements repeatedly is common.
- Some of the elements may be apparently missed out altogether or passed over so lightly that they appear insignificant by comparison with the others.
- Aspects of the process may be delayed for some people, until triggered by later events.

TEN ELEMENTS OF BEREAVEMENT

The 10 elements of bereavement are listed first and then considered a little more fully:

1. Shock	■ Numbness, protection from emotions, which might otherwise be overwhelming.
2. Acute grief	■ Raw, overwhelming sadness: compulsion to think about the loss despite the pain of doing so. ■ High arousal – the fight or flight response.
3. Defence mechanisms Denial	■ An optimism that may feel unreal: 'It is a release from their suffering so there is no need to be sad for them.' 'The person has gone to a better place, so I must be happy for them.' 'Maybe the person isn't really dead after all.'

Searching	■	Occasionally a physical search for the dead person; revisiting places associated with them.
Avoidance	■	Hyperactivity: too busy to allow painful feelings to surface.
Pretence and fantasy	■	Behaving as though the loss has not occurred.
	■	Prince Albert's shaving water continued to be put out daily after his death.
Bargaining	■	Often with God, regardless of faith or absence of it: 'Bring him back and I promise I will. . . .'

4. *Fear*
- Of violent emotions; of going mad; of an inability to cope.
- Often worse at night; vivid dreams and nightmares.

5. *Guilt*
- 'If I had/hadn't done X this would never have happened.'
- 'If only I had been a better friend/ colleague/partner/spouse. . . .'
- 'If only I hadn't quarrelled with her.'
- 'It's my fault.'

6. *Anger and resentment*
- With self, dead person, doctors, God, the boss, the company, heartless colleagues, etc.
- 'Why me?'
- Often (mis)directed onto those close to the bereaved.

7. *Depression*
- 'It's pretty miserable here without her.'
- 'Life has no meaning any more.'
- 'I wish I was dead too.'
- Withdrawal, apathy, lowering of standards, regression, emotional exhaustion.

8. *Loneliness*
- 'I've lost someone who saw the job the way I did: that's a rare thing – they're irreplaceable.'
- 'I feel so alone.'

9. *Resolution*
- Resignation/acceptance.
- Emotional energy withdrawn from the lost person, job, home, etc. and reinvested into the present and the future.

10. *Introjection*
- Internalising the qualities of the person who has died.

1. Shock

- Numbness, protection from emotions, which might otherwise be overwhelming.

Even when death is expected, its arrival usually comes as a shock, lasting from a few minutes to a few days. The function of shock is to enable us to carry on somehow for a limited time. It protects us from the full impact of what has happened, whether we have lost a limb in an accident or an emotional limb through the death of someone close to us.

Shock can be expressed in panic, numbness or a mixture of the two. The first leads to the hyperactivity that is well-suited to dealing with the practical arrangements associated with the aftermath of death, such as informing people, arrangements with funeral directors and the funeral itself. The second is the complete opposite: an apathy, which requires everyone else to do everything, including, if possible, looking after the bereaved person.

> Dick's mother phoned him at 6.30 a.m. to tell him that his father had just died from a heart attack. By 8.30 a.m. he was on his way to the other side of the country where his parents lived. He had already written a two page email to his secretary and put through a coherent ten minute phone call to his deputy unscrambling his plans and ensuring that essential work was undertaken in his absence. He was able to be relatively competent because his state of shock shielded him for the moment from the reality and emotional impact of what had happened.
>
> He did not feel anything very much, except for the adrenaline surge to get cracking fast. On one level, he did not really believe it had happened. He was conscious that he wanted to see his father's body to be sure. The shock acted like a protective blanket to prevent him being overwhelmed and incapacitated.

2. Acute grief

- Raw, overwhelming sadness: compulsion to think about the loss despite the pain of doing so.

- High arousal – the fight or flight response.

In 1999, six weeks after Stephanie Kugelman became chairperson and chief executive of Young & Rubicam's New York office, her husband Arthur died of complications related to lung cancer. She took a week off after his death and then returned to work. Mrs Kugelman had friends and family to give her comfort, but she felt that there was no one to talk to about her particular circumstances: dealing with grief and running a company. When she was consumed by emotion at the office, she would take a walk around the block to compose herself, but it was hard to maintain her attention span. 'You're reading something and not retaining it,' she said.[5]

Shock is usually penetrated, sometimes within minutes, by sharp, sudden waves of acute grief in which the bereaved person is in a state of high arousal and agitation. It is characterised by the 'fight or flight' response, which is also found in fear, anger and physical pain. This is a phase when the ability to function well at work, school or home is diminished to the point of being non-existent. The person is completely absorbed in what has happened, as the grief begins to spear its way through the protective blanket of shock to reveal intense yearning and longing. It has been described as feeling as if the dead person has been torn out of your body. It can be accompanied by a variety of physical symptoms, such as feeling cold and clammy, an increased heart rate, anorexia, nausea, 'butterflies' in the stomach, frequently passing urine, diarrhoea and insomnia. Moments as intense as this can recur many years after the person has died.

Although thinking about the death is acutely painful, the need to do so is compulsive, despite the pain. It is a time of raw sadness, of restlessness and often sleeplessness, and of the need to talk, reflect, rage and weep. When asleep or just waking, hallucinations and strange vivid dreams are not unusual. Acute grief can be very upsetting to be near, which is one reason why the bereaved are given a wide berth by some people.

Elizabeth Jennings wrote in 1967:[6]

Time does not heal.
It makes a half-stitched scar
That can be broken and you feel
Grief as total as in its first hour.

What typically changes is not its intensity but its continuity. At first the bereaved person may be constantly moving in and out of acute grief, but as the days or weeks pass, longer intervals will gradually elapse between being preoccupied with and pining for the deceased. But its power may feel as great when it does return. It is 'the heartbreak in the heart of things', as W.W. Gibson wrote, the potential price of any genuine friendship and love.

When the baby of a colleague died in tragic circumstances, Joan's own work suffered. When her manager talked through what was troubling her, falteringly she told him that she had lost a baby at the same age, five years before. She was particularly troubled because the incident had brought memories flooding back. A painful aspect of that had been her general practitioner telling her that she was grieving 'abnormally', because she was still so upset six months after the event. It was as if he had twisted a knife in the wound of her grief and added a further unnecessary burden to it. That word 'abnormal' had stuck in her throat ever since. She was torn between her anger at the insensitivity of the general practitioner and her sneaking suspicion that the doctor may have been right and she was 'abnormal' as well as desolate at the loss of the child she loved so intensely. Talking it through with her exceptional boss enabled her to re-evaluate the whole experience, and in doing so a degree of detoxification occurred for her.

3. Defence mechanisms

Denial

- An optimism that may feel unreal:

  'It is a release from their suffering so there is no need to be sad for them.'

  'The person has gone to a better place, so I must be happy for them.'

  'Maybe the person isn't really dead after all.'

The value of denial in bereavement is that it helps protect us from the necessity of coming to terms with all the pain at once. To register the reality of death at a deep level seems to involve the need to question the fact of it in a variety of ways. A few people cannot believe that the person has died. This is reinforced when the body has not been found or is not recoverable, so that the bereaved person cannot see it. Perhaps a mistake was made:

- I just can't believe that he really has gone.
- I keep thinking that he is going to walk through that door this evening just like he always has.
- I feel as if I'm going to wake up and find out that it was a bad dream after all.

Denial can also be reflected in vivid dreams, in which the dead person is alive again, or sometimes in waking dreams, in which the person's presence is felt, usually but not always invisibly.

A person may be helped to come to terms with the reality of death by seeing and spending time with the body, either at the undertaker's Chapel of Rest or hospital or by keeping the body at home. When my father died, his body stayed at home until the funeral so that members of the family could say their farewells in their own time, at their own pace. His body had to be removed temporarily for embalming so that it would not begin to decompose. In situations such as war, accidents or disasters where it is not possible to see the body, the bringing home of the remains in a coffin can be a real comfort and help the bereaved to move on in their process of mourning.

On the other hand, this does not apply universally, and some wish that they had not seen the person after death, especially if the body has been laid out badly with, for example, the mouth dropping open. A dead body soon looks, feels and smells unlike the person who has died, even shortly after death. So, those who have not seen the body of their loved one after death do not need to feel that they have missed something essential, as the arguments on this issue are often finely balanced.

Of course it is often not a matter of choice, for example, for the person who finds someone dead or is required by the police to identify the body of someone close to them.

A variation on the theme of denial is the acceptance of the fact of death, but a refusal to acknowledge the pain of bereavement, sometimes on the basis of religious belief.

> The mother of Liam and Beryl told them that they must not be sad about their young son, because he had passed on to be with Jesus. This piety felt so false to the mourning parents that it helped to break their links with the church for many years.

At work, the bereaved person's use of denial in thinking and talking only some of the time with only some people needs to be respected. Equally, it is not helpful to impose denial on the person because of everyone else's discomfort with what has happened. Striking the right balance requires awareness and sensitivity.

Denial can also be expressed through humour and behaviour that appears to take no or an inadequate account of the person's death. 'Gallows humour', as it is sometimes called, is a coping mechanism used by some in professions where death or dead bodies are familiar experiences. It can be shocking to an outsider but can help the person to get on with their job efficiently by distancing themselves from the person in the body. Surgeons may live quite a double life out of necessity in the way they relate to the anaesthetised body in the operating theatre and to the conscious person, who needs respectful, sensitive and empathic communication. They vary in how successfully they can make the switch.

> Rick, one of the computer programmers, committed suicide by hanging himself: he had a young family and money troubles. He had kept himself to himself, so his colleagues did not know him too well. The response of the majority was to express no sympathy but to see him as weak and stupid. One of his colleagues felt very differently, however, as his own brother had died in the same way two years before. He found it hard to come to terms with the lack of compassion in the others for the desperation Rick had obviously felt before he took such a step.

Searching

Searching, like most of the so-called stages, can be a layer of the bereavement process, which takes many different forms. Sometimes it takes the form of a physical search, such as visiting old haunts or the hospital or place where the death occurred, hoping in some strange way to find the deceased person there. A preoccupation with places, objects or memories associated with the person who has died, such as photographs, letters and possessions is characteristic of searching. Contact with old friends or family may all play their part in a kind of modern pilgrimage. Our efforts to rediscover in some way the person we have lost can also have a religious dimension.

Many who are newly bereaved seek out spiritualist churches or visit mediums in the hope of making contact with the deceased. An interest in a life after or beyond death need not, however, be dismissed as merely wishful thinking for victims of superstitious suggestibility. At such a time, we may be in a state of heightened sensitivity to dimensions of spiritual reality. It is also possible that there may be a bit of both.

The search for all the fragmented memories of the dead person helps to internalise them, so that they can be remembered in the inner world of the mind now that they no longer exist 'out there' and no longer exist only as an absence in the outer world. In an ancient myth, Isis searches the universe for the dismembered parts of Osiris in order to re-member him. Part of the search is to restore the other in memory, which can fade quickly, especially with someone with whom we have been very close.

In doing this, the bereaved may also be reconstructing themselves with a new identity or recovering their old one, and remaking their understanding of the world in which such an event has happened.

Avoidance

A common defence mechanism is to avoid thinking or talking about the loss. An effective way of achieving this is to become hyperactive, too busy to allow painful feelings to surface. So the person becomes preoccupied with other activities, either on quite a mundane level, such as maintaining home, garden and work, moving house or by taking on demanding new activities. They can insist on organising the funeral single-handedly and disposing of the deceased's belongings immediately, possibly to regret doing so later.

It can lead people to rush back to work too soon before they are really ready, and taking on new projects unnecessarily. The former can help counter the destabilising impact of grief, which means that extra care and concentration are required to be competent in everyday living, most especially activities that are potentially dangerous, such as driving.

At work it is important at least to consider whether a newly bereaved person can be given a break from such activities. In the shorter term, support and supervision may need to be stepped up. Whether this is done discreetly or openly will depend on the personalities and relationship with the bereaved person. They may need to be given shorter runs and encouraged to take things slowly and carefully, for the sake of others as well as themselves.

Pretence and fantasy

Denial is sometimes extended to the point of pretending that the person is not really dead. It can take many forms, such as talking aloud with the person as if he was alive, and maintaining his things in place, maybe even putting out clean clothes or laying a place at table for him. Queen Victoria is reputed to have ordered Prince Albert's shaving water to be put out daily after his death. Such pretence can play a useful, if intermittent, role in helping someone cope. Occasionally it becomes more prolonged and then, as with other defence mechanisms, it may block the grieving process if the person becomes stuck in this phase.

The accidental laying of an extra place at the meal table or other routines do not constitute pretence: they may just be forgetfulness. Imaginary conversations with the dead person can also be held in full awareness that they have died, and be a source of great comfort. Conversing with someone who has died can be a way of letting the relationship go more gradually and gently than the suddenness of death permits. It might also express a belief, conviction or hope that the person is in spirit not only still alive but also able to hear human words directed towards them. Behaviour tends to change at a slower pace than changes in our understanding or attitude.

Bargaining

A final example of a common defence mechanism is bargaining, which often has a deep psychological power, even if rationally we believe that nothing can be achieved. We may be drawn to try trading good behaviour, extra effort, prayer or personal sacrifice in the hope that the person may be contacted again, that perhaps the death was all a big mistake or, if it was not, then there may at least be contact with them beyond the grave.

The 1956 film *The Seventh Seal* by the Swedish filmmaker Ingmar Bergman was a vivid fantasy exploration of bargaining. In it, while plague ravages the countryside, a knight plays chess with death, who is depicted as an almost human figure and tells him that his time has come. The knight tries to bargain for just a little more time in which he hopes that he would be able to make sense of his life and its purpose before he dies. So long as the knight can keep the game going, so he can continue to live, although death warns him that 'I always win in the end'. The wish for just a little more time is a common human sentiment about death. Whether or not that happens seems to be as much a product of luck or the lack of it, as of careful, healthy or virtuous living.

4. Fear

C.S. Lewis opened his short book about the death of his wife, *A Grief Observed*: 'No-one ever told me how like fear grief is'.[7] There are many different fears associated with some bereavement, although few individuals are likely to experience them all. These include the fear of strong emotions, of going mad, of being alone in the house, of not surviving practically and/or emotionally without the deceased, of other people dying next or of following the deceased into illness and death.

Especially for those who have not been bereaved before, the experience can be frightening partly because it is so unfamiliar. Even if the bereaved do not feel that they are going mad, they can seem like strangers to themselves, reacting in a way they have not experienced before. Their usual sense of identity may feel lost or out of control as they are swept along by complex, swiftly changing and sometimes violent emotions. Their bond with the dead person can make them feel strange or alienated from other people. If others withdrawing from them reinforce this, the nightmare can intensify.

The nightmare can for some be literal. The dream sometimes involves the death or the deceased person coming back to life or living in another place.

> Mary dreamt that her mother had phoned to say she was living in a town 20 miles away, and wanted to see her new grandson. It stirred up some confusing and painful feelings for her, as her mother had died when she was a young child. Although she was now in her mid-twenties and happy with her partner, when Mary had become pregnant and her baby was born, she had missed her mother greatly. Her unconscious mind had brought out thoughts that she had no idea were lurking there. Supposing her mother had not died and was living elsewhere and was getting in touch? How wonderful, but then how could she have neglected Mary all these years?

So the dream brought out Mary's feelings of betrayal by her mother for dying, even though her rational mind knew that she could not be blamed for her terminal illness. So at a conscious level there was no room for her anxiety or anger. Dreams can play a powerful, fascinating and useful role in linking our unconscious to our conscious mind, because the rational mind, which sifts and censors, is off duty while we sleep. For Mary this dream was a frightening experience, but it also enabled her to experience some of her anger with her mother for dying, an anger that her conscious mind could not logically countenance. After all, her mother's death had been a tragedy for them both, which she knew rationally that her mother had fought hard to prevent.

What can also be unnerving about such dreams is that the bereaved may sometimes find it difficult to wake up from them and separate them clearly from waking 'reality'. It helps to share such dreams with someone who is trusted not to be alarmed, shocked or dismissive. Knowing that such experiences are not unusual in bereavement protects the dreamer from unnecessary fears of mental instability.

The violence of some of the feelings experienced in bereavement mirrors the violence implicit in death. Even the gentlest of deaths extinguishes the vital spark of life. Strong language reflects this: feeling 'torn', 'agonised', 'cut in two', 'tormented', 'tortured'. Fear is a very natural response to that kind of reality.

5. Guilt

Guilt is often an element in relationships between the living, so why should death remove it? The opportunities for guilt in bereavement pile up. There can be a host of regrets:

- Why didn't I spot his loss of weight?
- Why didn't I get her to see the doctor sooner?
- Why wasn't I more patient when he was ill?
- I could have done more to relieve her suffering, improved the quality of her life or even prevented her death.
- If I had known that this was going to happen, I would never have spoken to him like that: no wonder he was making so many mistakes those last few days.
- She was difficult to get on with, but I'll never forgive myself for not trying harder.

The sense of having done wrong to the person who has died is not uncommon among the bereaved. The idealisation of the dead person can stimulate even more guilt. Its underlying power often springs, however, from something even more fundamental: 'I am alive and he or she is dead.' That kind of guilt can persistently nag away, even though there may be absolutely no rational justification for it. The feeling for the value of life in the face of death cannot be minimised, although some religious beliefs may do so.

Being the one still alive can contaminate the simplest and most innocent of life's pleasures. 'It's all very well for me to enjoy this, but it's never again going to be possible for him to have a jar of real ale or strawberries and cream or listen to a Mozart symphony or watch Tottenham.'

> Carl's grandfather spoke at the eight-year-old boy's funeral, after his tragic drowning in a canal. 'I loved that boy so much. He was so full of life, but it would never have done to have told him so, because youngsters can get to think too much of themselves if you're not careful. But now I wish I had told him somehow how much I loved him.'

The importance of expressing appreciation, affection and respect at work and at home is often most poignantly realised when someone's death makes it no longer possible. Sometimes there is also the wish to have cleared something up or to have said something that now can never be said. Whatever the reality behind the guilt, the need to feel the guilt and regret, and then to undergo the experience of forgiving oneself and accepting one's limitations is a crucial part of grieving for some people.

In a poor relationship the guilt may be especially focused on the fact that we have run out of time to improve things. A sense of relief that the person is no longer around can also fuel guilt.

Lastly, guilt can interweave with or add to any of the other aspects of bereavement, such as depression, anger or fear. They may be thought of as self-indulgent, weak or sinful, depending on values, gender, culture and other conditioning. Bereavement sometimes takes the lid off powerful emotions that have hitherto, more or less, been successfully repressed.

> Simon grew up with the view that anger and aggression were wrong, and avoided fights as a child. He was known as a peaceful and peace-loving person. A drunken motorist then tragically killed his girlfriend, and he grieved deeply for her, but apparently without much anger. He would say dismissively: 'Of course I am angry but what is the use of dwelling on it. The poor sod that did this is bound at some level to be punished enough by the realisation of what he has done. Anyway, no amount of belly aching by me is going to bring her back again, so what is the point? Anyway, I have little right to feel bad compared to her: I have lost someone, sure, but she has lost everything'. Such feelings were a waste of time in his book.
> Then one evening Simon was having a drink with some friends, when a drunken youth started abusing him. His mind went blank at some point until he found himself being hauled off this lad, whom he had attacked so severely that he had to go to hospital. This incident was the trigger for him to seek further support through his personnel manager. Previously, Simon had reassured her that he was fine and was coping, despite some concern in the company that he seemed to be struggling to get back into the swing of work nearly a year after his girlfriend's death.

Fortunately, an understanding of the human response to loss can sometimes help us re-evaluate such a rejection of part of our feelings. Whatever our conditioning, we need the ability to feel without guilt, anger, depression and fear, in order to grieve.

6. Anger and resentment

- With self, the dead person, doctors, God, the boss, the company, heartless colleagues, etc.
- 'Why me?'
- Often (mis)directed onto those close to the bereaved.

Fury can be acted out in uncontrolled violence, leading to grievous bodily harm and murder, but it can also fuel and energise the fight for justice and a better world. Intrinsically, therefore, it is part of being human and needs to be understood, accepted, channelled and managed in a constructive way.

Anger is an integral part of most healthy grieving, even though it may be disguised. We can be angry on behalf of the person who has died for their loss of life and perhaps too for their suffering. Anger is, for many, a frightening emotion, either if it is being felt or someone else near is show-ing it. Consequently, supporting someone in their anger may feel alien, but bereaved people need to be helped to express it and appreciate that it is a normal part of most grieving. This is especially important if other people are trying to undermine it. The venting of anger, without physically hurting anyone, can be a valuable means of relieving accumulated stress.

Anger can feel very painful and be difficult to express. It can seem inappropriate and even shameful. It is sometimes difficult to find a suitable target for one's anger, although a target may present itself or be found through transferring feelings onto someone near at hand. Friends, colleagues, family or neighbours who gave less time than was needed; doctors, nurses, clergy or others in a caring role, who were inadequate or seemed so, can all become the object of anger. Annie Hargrave, a counsellor quoted in Chapter 1, wrote of an incident after the death of her 21-year-old son: 'My employer had sons of a similar age to mine and one of them popped in to see him unannounced one day. There was some mild banter, entertaining, and then I came out with an unprovoked cutting remark, which in psychoanalytic language would be described as an attack. I felt ashamed of myself and it told me there was a long way to go yet. If I could come out of the blue with an attack on someone for having a live son, I certainly had a while to wait and work to do before wholeness . . . and work'.[8] Not everyone is as self-aware as her or as stringent about her readiness to work again. That depends on the nature of the work, but it is as well to reflect on how easily it is to dump anger on inappropriate targets and how damaging it can be if the target is vulnerable and less powerful than we are.

An employer can also be the target of anger, if it is thought that work was the cause of death. That this may be part of the grieving response does not mean that there was no bullying or oppressive style of management operating. It is not acceptable to dismiss anger as just part of the grieving process as if that lets senior management off the hook of taking its cause seriously, irrespective of whether it is expressed formally in the form of a grievance or not.

> The new general manager (GM) came in to tighten the place up. A tough workaholic, who prided himself on his lack of sentimentality, he soon got to work on Jim, who was from the 'old school' of industrial relations: short on confrontation, long on building trust and two-way understanding. The GM assumed that Jim had been soft on the unions for many years and had conceded too much. Besides, he didn't like the way Jim usually left work at about 6 p.m. to be with his family or the youth club, to both of which he was devoted. Jim found it difficult to attend the GM's long evening meetings. He felt increasingly stressed with the unrelenting pressure from the GM. After 18 months of this, he was made redundant. A month later he became ill: a myeloma was diagnosed and he died six months later, aged 48. He took his illness with the same stoic forbearance with which he had struggled to tolerate and adjust to the GM's behaviour. His widow was aware that some cancer may be stress related. While a connection could not be proved, her anger sprang from her conviction that the GM had caused his death.

Members of staff bubbling over with rage have approached trades union representatives and human resource managers. Sometimes the fury may seem disproportionate to the incidents or behaviour that triggered it. Part of the skill that is required is to help the staff member cool down before helping them to decide whether pursuing the matter further is appropriate.

While anger is part of the bereavement process, it can also be a mask for grief, especially for those men conditioned to believe that anger is manly, whereas grief is not. Such men may need encouragement to express their underlying grief so that they can be purged of it. This applies in reverse. Some women have been brought up to think that anger is incompatible with femininity. They may unconsciously mask their resentment with grief and need help to acknowledge their anger directly and not only through tears.

Some resentment may be directed against the deceased person for dying, for not fighting harder, for leaving us to cope with so much. Although this anger may appear rational and consequently easier to admit in the case of suicide or carelessness, it can also be strongly felt where someone had no means of preventing their death. The question can still rumble away beneath the surface: did they really have to die, leaving us inadequately supported? Could they not have tried harder to fight death? This anger sometimes breaks the shell of our denial.

God may also become the focus of anger. Anger transcends superficial rationality in many ways: committed atheists can be as angry with the God they do not believe in as a more conventionally religious person. Innocent suffering is part of the human condition; as a result of natural and human disasters and the way diseases, crashes and collisions happen, people can still consequently be affronted with God when they or someone close to them becomes a victim. The religious tradition is full of the struggle to reconcile belief in a loving God with suffering. Somehow suffering has to be understood as part of the divine purpose, from which God does not escape. Atheists, with their own struggles, are glad to be off this particular hook.

Anger, whatever the target, is a natural, if uncomfortable, response to the death of someone we care about. It is important that we are allowed and indeed encouraged to own it, without it being undermined by intellectual analysis. When it is adequately expressed, we will usually come to understand which parts, if any, are rationally justified and which have been burned up in the fire of the moment.

Dylan Thomas[9] wrote in his poem:

Do not go gentle into that good night.
Old age should burn and rave at close of day;
Rage, rage against the dying of the light.

But the grief implicit in the anger finally bursts through:

Curse, bless me now with your fierce tears, I pray.

7. Depression

After the exhaustion of the earlier stages, bereavement often causes us to sink into depression: uncertainty, lack of confidence, apathy and despondency. It has been described as a condition in which everything and everyone seems grey. As one person put it: 'I lost the ability to see things in colour'. It can find expression in a desire to stay within the safety of our own home or with a few close friends and family. At work, we might withdraw from others, literally keeping our head down. Absenteeism from work, poor concentration and decline in competence are also common symptoms of the depression of grief can follow more obvious mourning. It often feels hard to stick close to people at this time, and colleagues may stimulate a strong and impatient urge to try to move the bereaved on before they are ready. The pressure on colleagues to maintain goodwill and tolerance with someone under-performing as well as output can be tough. If the bereaved person is off work, it may be possible to get temporary extra help. But if they have returned and are not firing on all cylinders, colleagues need to be willing, understanding and flexible if they are to play their part in helping the bereaved person back to full functioning. Those who are marked by scars, bandages, plaster or crutches inspire easier empathy than those with the invisible wound of a broken heart.

> Give sorrow words. The grief that does not speak
> Whispers the o'er fraught heart, and bids it break.

So, in *Macbeth*, Shakespeare suggests the heart of grief that finds expression, not in the agitated energy of acute grief, but in whispers. Instead of the unreal optimism of denial, there is the bleakness in which any flicker of light at the end of the dark tunnel is extinguished. Apathy, despondency and despair are characteristic of times in which the long-term implications of loss begin to be realised. The physical exhaustion in grief is most in evidence, lowering morale even more. Lack of energy makes it doubly hard to maintain standards at work or at home. Self-care and personal appearance may deteriorate. The depressed person is likely to contribute minimally to relationships and needs to become more of a 'taker' than a giver. All of this will be more or less difficult, depending on how different it is to their previous behaviour.

> 'Andy's partner died eight months ago and as his manager I made every allowance at the time. He seemed to be handling it well; but now I'm having second thoughts. He is pretty ungracious with everyone who supported him, and I am beginning to think that he is taking advantage of the situation and being a little too sorry for himself'. Andy's manager was making the common error that support for a bereaved colleague only needs to be relatively short term. Andy was still very much in the grip of grief and his behaviour gave all the indications of depression, a natural part of the process. It was important for his manager to

acknowledge that Andy's behaviour was atypical of him. It was an expression of some of his grief, which, with good support rather than censure, he was more likely to work through until he could function again in a way that his manager wanted.

This sadness can be even more confusing in those with a general tendency towards depression. For them, bereavement can add an extra layer of sadness, which may make it especially hard to endure. Support for them may therefore be doubly important, even though their behaviour when bereaved may seem to vary less from their norm than the behaviour of those not subject to depression.

There are, in any case, times when it can feel harder to support the bereaved, and consequently when they are particularly prone to feelings of 'being let down'. The drama of death can keep the adrenaline going on both sides at first. When that runs out, the longer haul of mourning and support begin.

Shirley wrote: 'I never lost anyone really close to me until my father died, just eleven months ago. I knew sadness and pain before then but never as great or as lasting as I know now. Slowly my optimism and self-confidence are coming back; I lost them when he died. I know I will never be the same person I was. It feels as if I have lost some of the magical power and strength he gave me simply by his being alive – I have lost something that I had simply by knowing he existed somewhere on this earth'. Shirley was a dynamic person at work with responsibility for supervising and managing a team of 20, as well as being a mother of two young children. She felt that her energy was a crucial part of her effectiveness at work and home, and struggled with the loss of it during the 18 months after her father's death. She felt she was letting other people down as she struggled to regain her sense of who she was.

8. Loneliness

- 'I've lost someone who saw the job the way I did: that's a rare thing – they're irreplaceable.'
- 'I feel so alone.

As the preoccupation with the dead person recedes, loneliness creeps in, especially for those left to live alone. Sexual loneliness sometimes leads to promiscuity and then to more guilt. In the earlier phases, there is a kind of emotional companionship, albeit painful, through the preoccupation with the one who has died. As this fades, the reality of life without the loved one becomes a further source of pain, as if the lonely heart of grief has been finally reached.

If the dead person was a living-in companion, there is a whole lifestyle to change. Everything previously undertaken together, from shopping and housework, to meals, weekends and holidays, must now be undertaken alone. The adjustment that is required is colossal, especially if they have been together for a long time. For some, such as some gay or lesbian couples, there is an added dimension to their pain, because their loss may not be accepted or even realised by others. Hence the crucial role gay support groups can play in this area.

The loneliness of those caring for a child or a disabled person, who subsequently dies, can also be especially intense. So much of the previous life had been taken up with care that the resulting gap and emptiness might feel huge.

Loneliness can also be felt sexually, sometimes as an increase in libido. This can feel like betraying the person who has died and be an added source of unnecessary shame, instead of reflecting how sex was a channel for expressing love and a good deal besides. Loneliness can often be most acute in bed.

> The most difficult hours were the ones before dawn. She slept with one arm over a pillow. Sometimes she nudged the pillow lightly with her elbow, her signal to Rustom that she wanted his arm around her. When the human weight did not materialise, she awakened to emptiness, relearning the emptiness of loss before the sunrise.[10]

This need for closeness with another person, driven by great emotional need and power, can bring the recently bereaved all too easily into close relationships, which do not have the sure foundation to last. There is likely to be an element of searching (see above), sometimes at the simplest level. The bereaved person finds him- or herself attracted to someone with characteristics that in some way remind them of the person who has died: for example the same coloured hair or background. The object of their affection can feel let down and second best, when they realise this: 'She was not really interested in me, but rather just looking for another him'. If the subsequent relationship breaks down, more complications are added to the recovery process.

The wise friend or colleague will therefore be as cautious as the wise bereaved person in moving into a sexual relationship. There is a need to acknowledge that the person who is still attached to the one who has died may not yet be emotionally (as opposed to legally) free to attach him- or herself to a new partner. The idea of clear sexual boundaries in relationships of various kinds can often be particularly helpful in bereavement.

The loneliness of the bereaved in other relationships should not be underestimated. When a wife dies, for example, the support can easily be concentrated on her husband: her teenage children's loss by comparison is sometimes virtually ignored. Instead, friends and family are tempted to lecture them on how they need to support their father.

> When Dad died last year I was 15 and lived most of my life with my mates; or thought I did. The strange thing was that no adult asked me how I felt, or said to me that they were sorry. It felt as if my relationship

with Dad didn't exist or was nothing compared to him and my mum. I suppose it wasn't worth mentioning. Yet they all seemed to expect me to support her.

9. Resolution

- Resignation/acceptance.
- Emotional energy withdrawn from the lost person, job, home, etc. and reinvested into the present and the future.

Resolution is not an end of love or memories or even the pain of missing the deceased. What it means is that painful feelings have been sufficiently worked through to free the bereaved person to live in the present and future, to function at or near their previous level. They are also hopefully able to develop the trust necessary to form new, perhaps even intimate, relationships. Some people, after a long partnership, cannot adjust and become stuck in depression. This is often linked to their feelings about their quality of life and a realisation that their own remaining time is too short for much of a new start, but that is not invariable.

> Gail was widowed, after a long marriage, in her mid-seventies and lived independently for a further 25 years. Despite various battles with ill health, they were by her own admission happy years. Although she thought of her marriage with pride, her husband had been dominating and demanding. For her being bereaved meant an element of sadness, but also of freedom to take charge of her own life. The small decisions gave her great pleasure: when and what to eat and how to order her days and nights.

The conclusion of the process is reached when the bereaved start to experience times when they feel, a little at least, as they did before. Joyce Grenfell writing in 1980[11] expressed the hope implicit in this stage in her poem:

> If I should go before the rest of you
> Break not a flower nor inscribe a stone.
> Nor when I'm gone speak in a Sunday voice.
> But be the usual selves that I have known.
> Weep if you must.
> Parting is hell.
> But life goes on.
> So sing as well.

There are, however, dangers in this stage of the process. The 'tyranny of positive thinking' can suggest unrealistic goals: with a stiff upper lip and plenty of denial, we might soon be living a normal life again almost as if nothing has happened. But there are no short cuts in grieving.

Bereavement can often be a tragedy, the quality of our survival depending on our working through the pain. The outcome may be peaceful acceptance for some, but sad or bitter resignation for others. It depends on many factors, including the level of independence in the relationship, the depth of affection, the quality of subsequent support and the meaning of death to the person affected.

10. Introjection

■   Internalising the qualities of the person who has died.

In a relationship, often the 'marital or relationship fit' finds expression in the different skills and knowledge that we each bring to our relationships of all kinds. So one may be a good cook or driver or first aider or manager of the household accounts or gardener and end up doing or at least supervising and leading the work needed in those areas within the relationship. If that person dies, the other one has to do the work himself or find another way of getting it done, unless that area is just to be neglected. Although the idea was originally expressed as that of 'marital fit', it might be better renamed 'relationship fit', as the process can operate in all kinds of close personal and working relationships, which are strengthened through a variety of complementary skills and attributes.

Distinctions drawn between working and personal relationships can be misleading. Though in relationships between the very young, play may dominate, there can be an unconscious work element, that of learning, which is their main task. Among older people, there is frequently a work task in so-called personal relationships, such as preparing a meal, creating a home or bringing up children. Equally in relationships at work, the bonding and friendship may be related but not restricted to a common task. Intimacy, usually not sexual, emerges in a relationship where people are working closely and intensely on a project. Of course, there are many examples of close relationships that are both 'personal' and 'working'. A celebrated example of this was that between the 20th century composer and conductor, Benjamin Britten, and his partner, the tenor Peter Pears.

What is sometimes called 'introjection' can help a bereaved person move forwards. In this (often unconscious) process, one member of a partnership internalises and perhaps acts out characteristics associated with the other. In absorbing the essence of the deceased, the bereaved person may take on some of their interests or even mannerisms. It operates at many levels: the husband who has never boiled an egg becomes a competent cook; the wife who has never paid a bill develops confidence in domestic finances. Where this happens, there is less danger of entering into an inappropriate second relationship as a means of getting a decent meal or escaping the anxiety of the unopened brown envelope. This process is not restricted to ex-partners. It is not unusual, for example, for an eldest child, especially of the same sex, to take on some aspects of the role of a deceased parent. So, an elder son (or daughter) may become more responsible, and perhaps take on some of his (or her) father's jobs around the house.

Introjection can also operate within a personality, although less obviously. A hitherto unsociable person develops socially after the death of their more outgoing partner, who previously 'covered that side of things'. Another person finds an interest in a subject in which their spouse had been knowledgeable.

Lily Pincus[12] put it: 'The mourning process involves the healing of a wound. Once the physical wound has been safely covered by healthy tissue, the process is completed and the patient does well to forget all about the injury. In mourning, however, the cause of the injury, the loss of an important person, must not be forgotten. Only when the lost person has been internalised and becomes part of the bereaved, a part which can be integrated with his own personality and enriches it, is the mourning process complete, and now the adjustment to a new life has to be made'.

BEREAVEMENT AND STRESS

There are parallels in the response to bereavement and to stress. It may help in supporting someone who is bereaved to keep an eye on how stressed they appear to be. Both stress and bereavement are naturally part of living a human life. Neither are intrinsically bad nor to be avoided. Equally, not everyone close to someone who dies becomes overstressed, but anyone may do, irrespective of the strength of character they may be assumed to have. How stressed they become can be in part due to the level of distress they experience at the loss of the person and the circumstances of their death. There may, however, be other factors, possibly unknown to people at work, such as what is going on in their life outside work in terms of loss and pressure. All of these things use up some of our reservoir of psychological and physical energy and resilience. The death of someone at work can stimulate the stress response in what may be for some a real sense of crisis. That response has been described in different ways. The following model is one way of charting how stress works.

The stress response

Alarm

Stage 1

Fight or flight: the body and brain prepare for action; people rally round with energy or disappear fast!

- speed up
- talk quickly
- move and walk faster
- eat and drink faster

Resistance

Stage 2

Fats, sugars and corticosteroids
are released for more energy

- irritability
- gastric symptoms
- tension
- insomnia

Exhaustion

Stage 3

Energy stores are used up

- 'cotton wool' head
- palpitations
- depression
- fatigue

If stress is building up in someone anyway, irrespective of a triggering event, such as a death at work, there are a number of ways in which it emerges: in the way we feel, the way we think, the way we behave and in the way our body reacts. Even though all of these four aspects of stress may be operating within an individual, one of the categories may be more obvious than the others. For example, some people's emotions are near the surface and it is seldom a mystery how they are feeling. Other people keep their feelings hidden, even perhaps from themselves and they are easier to know through their thinking. Others keep both their emotions and their thinking buried most of the time. They are doers but express themselves through their behaviour.

THE WAY THAT STRESS COMES OUT

If you are concerned about the level of stress a colleague or colleagues may be under, reflect on the four aspects of the way that stress may be experienced and expressed, as outlined in the model on the facing page. Like most models, it is not an exact description so should not be taken literally, but it is a useful description of tendencies and possibilities.

In crisis, as extra energy is released, people often have enough, even a surplus of resources, to be able to cope. Support from other people is often forthcoming, from work, home and friends, especially in the short term, until the crisis subsides. For some, however, support is thin; it is as if everyone else is reinforcing the stress rather than helping the person through it. Others might have good support available, which they refuse to or cannot access.

Feelings	Thinking	Possible behaviours	Bodily reactions
Angry	Confused	Drink too much	Constipation
Anxious	Defensive	Eat too much	Diarrhoea
Helpless	Forgetful	Restlessness	Dizziness
Irritable	Going round in circles	Sleeplessness	Heartburn
Worrying			Tight jaw
Nervous	Indecisive	Smoke too much	Heart rate increase
Miserable	Loss of concentration	Trembling	Hot and cold spells
Tired			Sweating
Panicky	Nightmares	Legs turn to jelly	
Tense			Muscle twitches
Not enjoying life			Rapid weight loss or gain

If the demands of the crisis continue, there is a danger of the psychological and physical energy getting used up and weariness builds up to the point where the person has little left. At that point, their ability to work effectively diminishes and collapses. With this kind of exhaustion a restful break, or some time off, so long as it is not spent in an equally stressful setting, can in itself lead towards recovery, although additional ways of dealing with stress may be essential and speed up the recovery process. These can include such things as counselling, exercise, healthy eating, meditation or relaxation exercises and massage. Any or all of these can be useful and valuable in the aftermath of a bereavement, as with any other experience that is stressful.

Notes

1 Tahmincioglu, E. (2004) 'Coping in grief, beyond "business as usual"', *The New York Times*, 1 February.
2 Parry, C. and Parry, W. (1994) *Tim: An Ordinary Boy*, London: Hodder and Stoughton.
3 Payne, S. (2004) *A Mother's Story*, London: Hodder and Stoughton.
4 Ellen, B. (2004) 'Death is not the end. I'll be with Sarah one day', *The Observer*, 23 May.
5 Tahmincioglu, E. (2004), *ibid.*
6 Whitaker, A. (ed) (1984) *All in the End is Harvest: An Anthology for Those Who Grieve*, London: Darton, Longman and Todd in association with CRUSE.

7 Lewis, C.S. (1961) *A Grief Observed*, London: Faber & Faber.
8 Hargrave, A. (2003) *Fit to Work*, Rugby: BACP in CPJ: Counselling and Psychotherapy Journal 3: 2003 March.
9 Thomas, D. (1952) *Collected Poems 1934–1952*, London: J.M. Dent & Sons.
10 Mistry, R. (1996) *A Fine Balance*, London: Faber and Faber.
11 Whitaker, A. (ed) (1984) *ibid*.
12 Pincus, L. (1976) *Death and the Family: The Importance of Mourning*, London: Faber and Faber.

Chapter 3

Children and young people

INTRODUCTION

The issue of children's bereavement is largely beyond the scope of this book, but this chapter is included for two reasons. Unresolved issues around childhood grief can often impact on us as adults, and may affect how we cope with our lives later on. This may lie behind why some people at work react to bereavement, apparently purely in the present, in a way that may seem even to them particularly puzzling. Secondly, for many adults it is all too easy to ignore or underestimate what children are going through after a death in the family or the death of a friend. Even in a relatively protected country, like the UK, about 1% of children are bereaved of a parent every year, that is about 135,000 children. It is estimated that 20 babies a day die at or soon after birth and 9,000 young people a year die before they reach the age of 14 as a result of illness or accident. Many of these young people have siblings. Sister Frances Dominica, the founder of pioneering a childrens' hospice in Oxford, subtitled her book based on that experience: 'Helping parents to do things their way when their child dies'.[1] That is an important principle of support for the grieving of any age, including, of course, children, as she makes clear.

Adults can easily feel confused about the grief of children, as if they inhabit a different emotional universe. What it was like to be a child can be quickly forgotten in the mists of time. What is more, they may have had no significant experience of grief when they were themselves young. Children, like their elders, are individuals and personalities vary. Parents may see similarities in their own and their son's or daughter's personality, but they quickly need to learn that they are not clones. Kahlil Gibran expressed it forcibly when he wrote:

> For they have their own thoughts.
> You may house their bodies but not their souls,
> For their souls dwell in the house of tomorrow,
> which you cannot visit, not even in your dreams.[2]

It is understandable that people want to protect children from the pain of grief as far as possible. They may also not wish to intrude inappropriately on their grief and do or say the wrong thing. So, avoidance can become a tempting strategy. The understanding of children about death can also be underestimated in order to protect the adults from being exposed to how they really feel. Furthermore, if those nearest to the child are themselves grieving, they may feel their emotional reserves are running dry and they have nothing left for the children.

The age when children are old enough to grieve continues to be a topic for debate. Dr. Dora Black of the Royal Free Hospital in London has undertaken pioneering work in supporting children who have witnessed such terrible crimes as the murder of their mother by their father. She uses a 'witness to violence' interview, similar to the debriefing interview for survivors of disasters. The drawings of children exposed to terrible experiences of violence leave no doubt as to the impact of that violence on them.[3, 4]

William Worden,[5] from his experience, including a study of 70 American grieving families and their children, concluded that children could mourn normally by the age of three or four, although others have argued that this capacity is not developed until adolescence. Dr. Naomi Richman, a child psychiatrist who has worked with children coping with war and violence, has argued that there is evidence that even younger children too young to speak are affected by witnessing violence: images can be remembered even at 18 months.[6]

John Bowlby argued that infants, coming to terms with the process of separation, experience grief reactions as young as six months. His studies included infants in hospital, at a time when it was common for parents to be kept away, even from visiting. The idea was that the appearance and departure of parents upset them, because they cried powerfully. Keep mothers, especially, away and the children stopped crying, often becoming listless and depressed although superficially easier for the staff to manage. Bowlby's work was influential in helping to change this practice to one of encouraging frequent and longer visits. Where possible, for very young children, a parent often now stays with them virtually all the time while they are in hospital. He demonstrated how deeply children can grieve at the loss, albeit temporarily, of the people on whom they most depend.[7]

As with adults, so with children there are many factors that bear down in different ways that influence the impact of a close bereavement on them. These factors may make the grieving even more difficult than it might have been anyway and be clues to the child who might need extra support to help them pull through:

- *The death itself* – if it was sudden and/or violent or even if it was unexpected for the child, because they were not prepared for it.
- *The person who has died* – if the deceased was the mainstay of their security – especially if he or she was a single parent; or if the child disliked or felt jealous of the bereaved; or if the child cannot speak of the person or idealises them or feels particularly guilty.
- *The surviving parent(s)* – if they lack support, are unemployed, have serious health difficulties of their own or are depressed. In such circumstances, they may be or become withdrawn and preoccupied with themselves to the detriment of their children or find it difficult to cope (as opposed to grieving strongly). That is also a source of added pressure on the child, especially if it is a sibling who has died.
- *The family* – the immediate or extended family, instead of being a resource to a bereaved child, is in some cases a source of further difficulty, with tensions, undue conflict or demanding siblings. On the other hand, the extended family that can be so important at such a time may be alienated or very remote.
- *The child himself or herself* – children, like adults, vary in personality and values and the degree to which they are able to access what support may be available. Any child will be helped in their ability to cope with their loss if they have the right kind of self-confidence, a sense of being respected, admired and loved for themselves rather than their achievements or strengths, ideally by their family, peer group and teachers.

CHILDREN'S GRIEF

How children grieve will be strongly influenced by their age and stage of emotional development. Adults supporting children should, therefore, be even more careful not to make assumptions about what they may be feeling than they would with adults. That is particularly important if the adult is a parent or someone else very close to the child, who may be more tempted to think that they know what the child is going through. Listening sensitively, but not too intrusively, to pick up clues in the child's behaviour as well as what they say is crucial in providing support.

Young children are naturally egotistical and feel that they are the centres of their world. Part of growing up is to become increasingly aware that this is not the case and that they do not have control or responsibility for all that goes on around them. This egotism impacts on their grieving process, in that it is not uncommon for them to be burdened by an unreasonable strand of guilt if a parent, sibling or someone else close to them dies or is killed. They can feel personally responsible for all kinds of reasons, for example if they had a row with the deceased, they did not love them well enough or think that they are being punished with their death for some reason. That reason may not be directly to do with the person who has died at all: for example, they may have been misbehaving or thinking hateful thoughts about someone. In supporting children, others need to be alert to this possibility of some such guilt, which can be directly addressed.

> When Sarah was 13, she had a row with her mother at breakfast. They did not part on good terms. Tragically, her mother was injured in an accident on the way home from work. Sarah was told of the accident by a friend of the family, but given no opportunity to visit her mother in hospital. Her father was in the hospital most of the time, but seemed to avoid her when he did come home. A week later, the same friend told Sarah that her mother had died, but her father never got round to talking with her about it. She was also not given the opportunity to attend the funeral. Ten years later, a personal crisis catapulted her into a need to talk through how she still felt about the tragedy. She felt that her partner's stiff upper lip mirrored her father's failure to give her any support at the time she most needed it and him. She retained a sense that men in her life failed to be concerned about how she really felt about painful issues. Her partner caught some of the unresolved anger towards her father, an important complicating factor when they started to unravel the communication issues between the two of them in the present.

SCHOOL

School is the workplace for many children, with similar issues facing teachers as managers. They also have to strive for the balance between crowding or intruding upon a bereaved child or one with a terminally ill parent or sibling and, on the other hand, failing to acknowledge the loss. In one school, a 5th form girl's father had died two months earlier. When she came back, nobody in the school mentioned it. It is important that the child is reassured sensitively that the opportunity is available for them to talk to someone they trust and who is trustworthy.

With children, especially younger ones, there are four common strategies adopted by adults: distraction, ignoring, reassurance and empathy, of which empathy is the most important. Some teachers still seem, however, only to have the first three in their repertoire. It's not always easy to distinguish between a child who is mildly upset or dramatising their feelings and one who is really upset. But the many empathic teachers notice the non-verbal and verbal clues as to how a bereaved child is really feeling and, as with a good manager (see Chapter 14), really listen with respect and humanity to them, and by doing so discern their needs and wants. Distraction and ignoring are options to be used sparingly, not invariably or without considerable care.

Before a pupil returns after the death of a family member, their teacher can sometimes usefully talk with the class about how they might feel returning to school in those circumstances, preparing to get the balance as right as possible between a continual stream of sympathy and ignoring them completely. The latter is a common problem, in those schools where the culture of denial is strong. Peer conformity is also an inevitable factor among young people, and to be bereaved is not conforming to most norms in British schools. Where there is a more public tragedy and the culture affirms mourning, children can be remarkably able in both grieving at school and also in supporting each other. Teachers need also to be vigilant for a sign that the vulnerability of bereavement does not becomes a magnet for bullying.

The peer culture and conditioning of boys tends to make it less easy for them to articulate how they feel, other than in coded ways, although their experience and depth of feelings, including grief, are no less real than those of girls.[8]

After the tragic death of a young mother recently, I was asked to assist the teacher in talking with the children before her daughter returned to school. We asked the class to imagine in pairs or three's how she might be feeling. This group of 10-year-olds identified virtually all the factors considered in Chapter 2, in as comprehensive a way as might be expected of most adult groups. When in the light of that, we asked them to consider together how they wanted to behave when she returned, the balance of concern and sympathy mixed with some judicious ignoring was striking. Her return had been helped by several text messages of sympathy and affection from some of her friends, especially but not only the girls. As in any workplace, the option of a short visit before she returned full time after the funeral was offered and accepted. She had some one-to-one time with the teacher at the end of a school day after breaking the ice with her classmates.

SAYING GOODBYE

A parent who knows that they are terminally ill may want to write letters, or notes, or put together a scrapbook for the child or children they are to leave behind. As the technology becomes available, they may want to express themselves on video to communicate what they sounded and looked like. As inadequate as these inevitably feel and as heart breaking to do, they can be treasured later. The parent needs to imagine at what age or even ages they are trying to communicate with their child, although that is secondary. The letters are likely to valued at different ages as the child, now grown up, puts themselves in the shoes of the parent struggling to write such an incredibly difficult letter.

Some people are helped by preparing for the death of someone close to them while they are dying, but children, especially younger ones, are less likely to be aware of terminal illness than adults, unless they are informed sensitively about what is going on. If that does not happen, they can be very upset or bitter later that they were not given the opportunity of saying their goodbyes, asking questions of the person while it was still possible or even just saying how much they loved them.

Children and parent may want to think about what kind of things they want to say to each other. Expressing their appreciation and love of each other, forgiveness for the quarrels or fights they have had, or asking each other questions, before it is too late, that they have been meaning to ask but have not got round to asking can all be on the agenda. If that opportunity is missed it can be a source of great and ongoing painful regret afterwards. Sometimes they can be supported to create that opportunity, rather than forlornly hoping it will just happen.

When it is a child who is dying, Claudia Jewett expresses the experience of many when she wrote:

> Even when children have an intuitive sense of their own impending death, they may be reluctant or afraid to bring it up because they don't want to upset their parents. And so the child faces the unknown, anxious and alone. Both caregivers and child wait for the other to indicate a readiness to talk about what is happening. When the topic does come up, it is not unusual for the dying child to be visibly relieved to have permission finally to ask questions and to receive the parents' reassurances and support.[9]

THE MEANING OF DEATH

Death has different meanings for children, as it does for adults (see Chapter 5), depending on their experience, culture and beliefs and the beliefs of those around them. At first the idea that the dead person exists some-where else makes some sense to the child, hence the importance of the idea of heaven as a physical reality. Before Copernicus and his followers made such a concept incredible for most people, religious and irreligious, there was the possibility of the adult view of death in many countries equating with that of the child. In general, separation for young children is the primary pain, whereas the finality of death may dawn on them slowly to the point, some into their teens, before they realise that death is both inevitable and inescapable for us all.

The meaning of death also depends for children on its familiarity. In most developing countries or especially places where there are wars or natural disasters, children at an early age are likely to see people who have died. In such circumstances, illusions about what happens to a body after death do not last long. The mystery and questions about what happens – if anything – to the person's spirit, of course, remain.

In many so-called developed countries in Europe and North America, for example, modern medicine and the death taboo mean that most children have little contact with the dying or are unlikely to see dead bodies. Furthermore, some of the basic facts can be kept from them in such a way that, if they discover them for themselves, can be the more frightening. Even though in stories, film and television, they are exposed to images of death, many children become sophisticated at distinguishing between fact and fiction. If it is the latter, it can be thought of as 'not real'. It is a game, entertainment. As play is a major and universal way that children of all ages both enjoy themselves and also learn, games involving killing and death can be experienced as fun and exciting. When some children are exposed to the real thing, it can be a massive jolt.

YOUNG PEOPLE AND MOURNING

When children lose someone close to them and if that is exacerbated by their exclusion from the mourning process, they may carry some unresolved grief into adulthood, which reinforces the intensity of their experience of loss later in life. To make matters worse, a child is sometimes made to feel, especially if they have reached adolescence, that their loss of a parent is secondary to the surviving parent's loss of a spouse. So they may be expected to support the latter and deny their own loss, especially if everybody else seems to be doing so around them.

While teenagers, especially boys, may be expected to be strong for others in the family, their own bereavement is hardly acknowledged. The idea may be floating under the surface that young people have had most of the crucial parenting by the time they hit the teens. Now they can appear closer to their peer group than parents and are looking away from the family for the focus of their life. So even they can underestimate their loss, but good parental support is a more than useful ingredient in making a good transition into adult life. The teenager who loses a parent is losing the chance of sharing with them all the triumphs, experiences, milestones, difficulties and crises in the rest of their life, as well as some of the battles, debates and arguments that herald growing independence.

If children have not reached adolescence, their grief may be ignored for a different reason. They are, perhaps, thought to be too young to cope with addressing it or perhaps to be upset by bereavement. Acknowledging it is thought to only make it worse.

A surviving parent needs to go through their own mourning but also to find ways of sharing some of that with their children. Giving children the attention that they need at this time may be difficult but it is essential that they do receive it. If possible it needs to come to a considerable degree from a surviving parent. The quality of extended family or community support is also very important, from grandparents, aunts and uncles, neighbours or friends, whoever is close to them and caring.

When Ian's wife died leaving him with a six-year-old son, elderly neighbours took on an unofficial grandparenting role and became a rock of care for the boy, constantly playing with him and giving him tea when he came home from school. Though there was no flexitime system at Ian's work, that did not stop his manager, Angus, suggesting to Ian that he come in late two or three days a week so that he could take his son to school. Angus had made the suggestion, because he touched base regularly with Ian enough to know 'how it was going'. This checking out was focused and did not take a great deal of time, maybe half an hour or less a week on average. Angus was in no doubt that that time was part of his managerial responsibilities, not an optional extra because he had a kind heart. At a time like this especially, Angus wanted Ian to be as successful a salesman as possible, but not at the expense of being a good father. He knew that Ian's enthusiasm and motivation would only be undermined if he was worried more than necessary about his son's welfare. Ian was largely free of divided loyalties, because of the level of support that he received at work.

Whether loss is acknowledged for young people may depend on the nature of the relationship. So a parent's death can be seen as very sad, while they may be expected to take that of an aunt or uncle in their stride, irrespective of how close the person may have been. Aunts, uncles, cousins and many other members of the extended family can be remote or close to the young person, whose grieving may vary accordingly. At times, such hierarchies are institutionalised for young people as well as for people at work. So, for example, in a British young offenders unit, the inmates may be allowed to attend the funeral of a parent or sibling, but not a grandparent. In some cases, however, the inadequacy of the relationship with their parents may be a contributing factor to them being inside. Grandparents can be the adults to whom they feel closest. In one such unit, Onley, near Rugby, an imaginative chaplain offered a service in the chapel at the same time as the funeral, when such a grandparent could be remembered and honoured.

Daniel is an industrial relations manager in the motor industry, whose story is described more fully elsewhere. After his father had left, he had lived with his younger sister and his mother, who when Daniel was 13 had collapsed in front of him, was rushed into hospital (after he alerted a neighbour) and died a week later. A few hours after her death, he was summoned to the hospital. There a priest, whom he did not know, told him that she had died. Daniel was then directed by the priest to kiss her and to go and tell his younger brother this terrifying news. Neither the priest nor anyone else apparently enabled him to talk about what was going on, to ask questions or to say how he felt. Like so many children in this situation, Daniel was locked into isolation by the insensitivity of the adult world. He was told to kiss his mother without warning or an explanation of how cold her body would be.

When we die, our body normally becomes naturally cold within an hour or so, but Daniel was experiencing the unnatural cold of a refrigerated body, which can shock people of any age if they are not prepared for it. We experience each other through all our senses, but touch is especially important in intimate relationships, such as that of a mother and child. Children need to be warned gently that the dead body of a parent may feel, smell, as well as look different, to the very familiar person when alive. When some of the feelings and smells are artificial to prevent the body from decomposing, it is an added complication to being with the body of someone who has died.

VIEWING THE BODY

For children as much as adults, seeing the body can help understand some of the reality of death, although care needs to be taken in case the person appears to look odd. Some explanation may be needed. Sensitivity is needed in explaining what the person looks like. Sometimes the body is made up to look even more unnatural than if they had been left more or less alone. I was with my mother when she died, and after a few minutes I drove to my sister's home to collect my family to come and pay their respects. It took me an hour or so, but when we got back, my mother's jaw had not been closed and had in death dropped open, making her look somewhat peculiar. My young boys, aged three and five, were not put out, however, and took it in their stride. One of them asked: 'I wonder what Grandma was saying when she died'.

Children are often mistakenly kept away from the funeral and feel it keenly later, although attitudes may be changing. When Virginia Ironside focused on the question 'Can a small child cope with a funeral?' in her column in *The Times* newspaper, 'scores of readers wrote in, many still smarting from being denied the chance when they were young to attend the funeral of a much-loved relative'. One of them, William Mathieson, who grew up in Liverpool in the 20s and 30s when the mortality rate among children was high, said that then 'it was common practice to lay out the bodies of children and adults in the front parlour. The front door of the house was left open and children and neighbours were free to go in at any time to view the corpse. I cannot recall any child being upset by this practice'.[10]

THE FUNERAL

The purposes of the funeral (see Chapter 10) do not only apply to adults. At the very least children should be given good information about the purpose of the funeral and what will take place, before being given the choice of whether to attend or not or encouraged to do so. In the case of a funeral of a parent or sibling, even though attending may feel like an ordeal, being left out of it may be worse, especially in the longer run. Being at (or even taking a part in) the funeral is a way of the importance of their relationship with the deceased being recognised and for them to honour them and continue the process of acknowledging that they have died. It also can give them a sense that others also cared about the one they loved.

The child's flowers or wreath should be given prominence on the coffin. They may also want to include symbolically a note, a drawing or momento in the coffin. It is important to ensure that their understanding that the person is no longer in the body is reinforced before and perhaps also at the funeral before it disappears for cremation or is lowered into the ground for burial.

> In William Worden's study[11] of 125 bereaved American children, between the ages of 6 and 17, 95% of them attended the funeral. In most families there was very little discussion about whether or not to include the children in this ritual. It was generally assumed that they would be there and they were. Children were included in the funeral planning and in the funeral itself in various ways. Being included also helped children to feel important and useful when many were feeling overwhelmed. A 10-year-old boy who helped carry his father's coffin said: 'It was kinda heavy but it felt good to carry his coffin'. Generally it was a positive experience, but the quality of preparation of the children for the funeral was important.

Human beings are social animals and experience grief both individually and collectively. Even though the funeral is a tough occasion, even for some an ordeal to be dreaded, it is also a time where the isolation of grief is permeated and perhaps diluted a little by being part of a shared experience. Preventing young people from coming to the funeral can reinforce the isolation that they can so easily feel, as easily as adults, if not more so, in grief.

CHILDREN OF A PARENT WHO HAS COMMITTED SUICIDE

If the parent was seriously or terminally ill, feelings may surface that they were robbed of a few days, weeks, months or years of their company, although it may be easier to accept than in other cases. It is difficult to reassure a child easily that they are not to blame and that the person did not want to leave them, in the case of suicide. The child will need to explore the reasons for such a drastic act, and their own feelings about it. They may feel guilty, sad, frightened and angry with the parent.

If they think of their parent as mentally ill, it can reinforce the fear that they may one day take the same path. On the other hand, if they regard them as not especially disturbed, they may feel desolate at the apparent lack of care or love that allowed them to act in a way in which their own needs were so apparently disregarded.

Where suicide was triggered by despair or acute depression, at some stage they may need to think through the alternative options that their parent did not take, on the basis that other such options will be available to them later in life (see also Chapter 9). Suicide is unlikely to be their only choice in the face of adversity. So they will not have to follow in their footsteps on this one.

> When Alex was 12, his father committed suicide, leaving him feeling stricken, guilty and bewildered. As the only son, he felt that if his relationship with his father had been better, it would not have happened. There was no note left and he had to cope with his transition into manhood without a close male role model nor a father with whom to talk things over. His mother seemed too distraught to take an interest in him or listen to how he felt. Alex ploughed a very lonely furrow for the next 10 years. After that his life took on a new direction: marriage, his own family and a good job following academic success at university. When he was made redundant in his thirties, however, after a successful career for 15 years, Alex had a crisis of confidence in which all the questions around his father's death resurfaced, as if it had happened only recently. The job search needed to be postponed for a while until he had worked through and recovered from some of the grief that had been on hold.

SUPPORTING EACH OTHER

There are a number of local initiatives, such as support groups, organised by different agencies, to help young people support each other. One project, for example, initiated a newsletter for bereaved teenagers. In one issue, Rachel, aged 14, wrote of her experience of living with her mother's cancer since she was 10:

> My mum is still alive at the moment, although nobody knows for how long – two months or two years. Even the doctors don't know. I was given four pieces of advice: (1) keep your chin up; (2) don't bottle things up; (3) it's nobody's fault; and the most important (4) live life to the full, every day is a new experience.

Lulu, aged 16, wrote of her mother's death three years before:

> I can't imagine her being dead. I don't really believe in heaven, so where is she? I can't understand how a person who was here so very alive can now be nowhere. I know we all die some day and death is reality – but I can't envisage it. I miss her each day, because as time goes on it's longer since I last saw her, last spoke to her in the flesh. I miss her to the point that sometimes I think I am going crazy needing to tell her all the things I never told her when she was here. Maybe I just never believed something like this would ever happen.

An 18-year-old wrote on the death of his father two years before:

> I feel like his death is partly my fault, and that I never got the chance to know him because I don't really talk and my dad wasn't a talker either. I know that I am going to miss him doing father–son things in future because my dad was always there when I wanted him . . . . I still cry, but I try not to in front of my mum, who is going through hell at the minute, and I try to be strong for her.

One teenager wrote of her thoughts from her mother's perspective shortly after the latter had died:

> I don't mind.
> I was never like the rest of you,
> Making plans about the
> Great things I'd do.
> I never thought of myself as much.
> You were the ones going ahead,
> Always, always running off without me.
> Now I am the one going ahead – to heaven,
> I am not afraid.
> If God wants me with him
> Then who am I to know better?

A checklist for supporting bereaved children and young people is on page 228.

FURTHER RESOURCES

The Child Bereavement Network
Telephone: 0115 911 8070
Email: cbn@ncb.org.uk

A national resource for bereaved children, young people, their families and other care givers.

The Child Bereavement Trust
Aston House, West Wycombe, High Wycombe, Bucks HP14 3AG
Telephone: Administrative: 01494 446 648 Information and support: 0845 357 1000
Email: enquiries@childbereavement.org.uk
www.childbereavement.org.uk

Launched in 1994, provides support, information and training.

CRUSE Bereavement Care

CRUSE House, 126 Sheen Road, Richmond, Surrey TW9 1UR
Telephone: Administration 020 8939 9530 Helpline 0870 167 1677
Email: helpline@crusebereavementcare.org.uk
www.crusebereavementcare.org.uk

Provides a list of publications for all age groups and local support and information. For local UK branch information, contact CRUSE nationally.

Winston's Wish

Telephone: 0845 203 040 5
www.winsonswish.org.uk

Founded in 1992 to help bereaved children and young people rebuild their lives after a family death, offering practical support and guidance to families, to professionals and to anyone concerned about a grieving child.

Notes

1 Dominica, Sister Frances (1997) *Just My Reflection: Helping Parents To Do Things Their Way When Their Child Dies*, London: DLT.
2 Gibran, K. (1926) *The Prophet*, London: William Heinemann.
3 Mesaud, C. (1992) 'Children who have seen too much', *The Guardian*, 15 April.
4 Black, D. et al (1993) *Father Kills Mother: Post-Traumatic Stress Disorder in the Children*, London: Cruse Bereavement Care.
5 Worden, W. (1996) *Children and Grief*, New York and London: Guildford Press.
6 Gill, L. (1992) 'Growing up after Tragedy', *The Times*, 18 August.
7 Bowlby, J. (1980) *Attachment and Loss: Loss, Sadness and Depression*, New York, NY: Basic Books.
8 Miedzian, M. (1991) *Boys will be Boys: Breaking the Link between Masculinity and Violence*, London: Virago.
9 Jewett, C. (1982) *Helping Children Cope with Separation and Loss: Childcare Policy and Practice*, London: B.T. Batsford.
10 Ironside, V. (1994) 'Finding a Friend in Death', *The Times*, 1 September.
11 Worden, W. (1996), *ibid.*

Chapter 4

Bereavement counselling

- What is bereavement counselling?
- Why bereavement counselling?
- How to start
- Timing

It has been estimated by Michael Reddy[1] that 80% of British companies use some form of workplace counselling. A particularly strong trend in recent years is that of Employee Assistance Programmes,[2] which give staff access to counsellors anonymously on a self-referral basis, normally for a limited number of sessions, varying from four to 12.

There is a paradox about counselling. On the one hand, it is based on good, 'normal', human communication at its best, a process many of us undertake when we are functioning well. On the other hand, the experience of it can feel very different from the rest of our communications. This is because, for many of us, it is relatively rare to be on the receiving end of high-quality, active listening, even though we benefit enormously from it. The value of being a client is reinforced by the time and attention being near 100% for the client and their needs. It can be simultaneously both ordinary and unusual, simple and highly skilled. Nowhere is this more evident than in dealing with death and bereavement.

WHAT IS BEREAVEMENT COUNSELLING?

In many bereavements, what counts most, and what is most needed, is quality support from friends, family and colleagues. If this is good enough, it will reflect consciously or unconsciously the skills of counselling, which underpin this book. But the words 'counselling' and 'client' will probably never be used, nor need to be. Where counselling differs from such support is not primarily in its content but in its context.

- *Contract* – The counsellor is not only discreet, but will have an explicit contract of confidentiality and time, which enhances the feeling of safety for the bereaved person (or client).
- *Independence* – The counsellor is normally outside the close circle of the client's acquaintances. The client is therefore likely to feel less responsibility for reassuring the counsellor that they are fine and coping well. There is often a great deal of subtle pressure on the bereaved to avoid sharing painful feelings honestly and thereby perhaps upsetting family, friends and colleagues, who may also be finding it difficult to cope. Although the sharing of grief can be crucially important for the future relationship of two people bereaved together, as for example with parents after the death of a child, the social pressure not to share deeply is frequently enormous.
- *Purpose* – The counsellor's task is to encourage the client to share the facts and the pain of the bereavement with a view to helping them to deal with it and any 'unfinished business' or other issues emerging. The sole reason for the counsellor and client to meet is in order to facilitate this. In the counselling session there are no interruptions or other distracting agenda to get in the way.

Although these three elements are more explicit in bereavement counselling, they are implicitly important in all bereavement support. A colleague or family member, for example, is clearly not outside the bereaved person's circle. However, they can, with skill, communicate the kind of emotional independence that frees the other person to do what they need to do or say what they need to say, rather than feel they have to take care of their supporter's feelings.

WHY BEREAVEMENT COUNSELLING?

There are a variety of circumstances in which bereavement counselling can be especially helpful and these include:

Inability to express/work through grief

The bereaved person may not feel able to express and work through their grief, due to its power and possibly the mistaken conditioning that to do so is self-indulgent, weak, counter-productive or a mixture of all three. (In such an instance, the person may become 'stuck' in one of the elements of bereavement, for example, depression or anger.)

Isolation

The bereaved person may be isolated without close, supportive relationships. They may live alone, keep themselves to themselves and have no relatives living nearby. Alternatively, these close relationships do exist with a network of friends and family, but the taboo on sharing real feelings, when they are painful, is so strong, with great embarrassment if the taboo is breached.

Trauma

The nature of the bereavement may itself have been especially traumatic, for example:

- in the death of a child or younger person;
- where dying has been particularly prolonged, painful or disfiguring;
- where it was thought to be avoidable;
- where it was especially sudden, as in an accident or an attack;
- where it was cumulative (when several deaths come close together or at the same time, as in war, a major incident or disaster);
- suicide.

Because depth of feeling is such a subtle and varied component of a relationship, it is impossible to offer objective criteria: a subjective assessment is more realistic.

> Grace's boyfriend was killed in a plane crash on a business trip. The wrong body was sent back and his real body was never found. She was a valued design engineer and her company were concerned to support her as well as they could. They arranged for some bereavement counselling. She felt that it helped her, not least to understand the powerful, grieving process through which she was going, and to keep her emotional bearings. What she found frightening was that for the first time that she could remember, her temper had got quite out of control on two occasions when there was no apparent link with her boyfriend's death. Her counsellor helped her acknowledge and express the anger in her grief, and understand the connections between her loss and her behaviour. Anger in bereavement was considered further in Chapter 2.

Work pressures

If there are changes and other pressures and stresses at work already, a bereavement may stretch an individual's emotional resources too far. By putting back some much needed extra support, counselling may help to restore the emotional bank balance. In the case of Grace, her personnel director had two aims. One was to care for a person in a very vulnerable state, the other – more hard-nosed but as legitimate – was to maintain the level of her contribution to the company as far and as quickly as possible. It is hardly surprising that she had not been her 'old self' since the tragedy.

HOW TO START

If external assistance may be helpful, the appropriate line or human resources manager should consult (via the company bereavement adviser if one exists) a counsellor or a suitable counselling organisation, such as those listed in Appendix 4, about the options open to the company. In doing so, it may be helpful to find out what code of ethics they subscribe to, such as that of the British Association for Counselling and Psychotherapy. It is customary to agree at the outset a budget ceiling for the maximum number of sessions or for the fee. This may be finalised after the first session, when the counsellor can better estimate with the client the length of time that may be needed. Most employee assistance programmes offer between four and 10 sessions. Six is commonly used by a number of organisations. Ideally, the norm should not be applied rigidly, but underlines a sense that long-term counselling is not usually funded by the employer. An exception to this is likely to be a bereavement that has been caused by or through work, irrespective of liability.

Alternatively, the bereaved member of staff could be given information about options, such as help from a local branch of Cruse Bereavement Care, and supported to make the initial approach independently. But it is worth remembering that at such a time, it is often best if the groundwork is done by another person. There can also be an advantage in having a small group of people in the company who have been trained in bereavement counselling or support. One of them can provide support to the staff member or his or her manager, and can perhaps help the bereaved person decide whether it is appropriate to seek further, external assistance.

Some organisations specialising in a particular cause of death, such as cot death, stillbirths, road traffic accidents and suicide, are among those listed in Appendix 4. To lose someone close to you through such a cause can be bewildering and feel isolating, with a sense that you know so little about it, compared to experts, who may be remote or inaccessible. For some people, to have access to sources of help and self-help, information and mutual support can be extremely important.

TIMING

Bereavement counselling, when it is appropriate, is often helpful a few months after a bereavement or even a year or so after, when immediate support is fading. The bereaved person may be going through a process of grieving, as described in Chapters 1 and 2, but start to find that there are issues that are still overwhelming or aspects of the bereavement that have not been addressed.

If the person finds that their return to some kind of normality at work and in other aspects of their life is painfully elusive, they may decide that counselling is worth trying. One person was referred by her human resources director to a counsellor, for example, a year after losing her partner in an accident. Another young man referred himself to a counsellor five years after his bereavement, when he finally admitted to himself that he was hopelessly stuck in trying to relate to members of the opposite sex, as if they had to become a clone of his late wife. However, after a traumatic experience, a counselling-based debriefing is likely to be desirable within a day or two. This is discussed further in Chapter 16.

Notes

1   Reddy, M. (ed) (1993) *EAPs and Counselling Provision in UK Organisations*, Milton Keynes: Independent Counselling and Advisory Service.
2   Feltham, C. (ed) (1997) *The Gains of Listening: Perspectives on Counselling at Work*, Buckingham: The Open University Press.

Section 2

Facing death

Chapter 5

What is death and what does it mean?

- Introduction
- Death and modern society
- Diversity of beliefs
- What happens when we die?
- Some personal thoughts about the meaning of death
- Rita and her gift through death

INTRODUCTION

In contrast with their forebears, many in richer countries live well into adulthood before death intrudes into their lives. Although we share with other creatures the fact that we die, the human imagination enables us to envisage death as well as life. Many of our dreams, visions, hopes, fears, anxieties and plans are linked to the fact that we die, as well sometimes as the fantasy that just perhaps we won't.

But we also live in the present. The experience of being alive – both pleasure and pain – can so concentrate our energy and attention on the present moment that it can feel as if death is something that happens only to other people. Kay Walker, a hospice counsellor and broadcaster, has described poignantly how her memories of the loss of a loved one felt for her as a child growing up in Trinidad.

> What matters?
> Very little, only. . . .
> the flicker of light   within the darkness,
> the feeling of warmth   within the cold,
> the knowledge of love   within the void.

Death itself can be thought of as both a passive and an active force. In Ingmar Bergman's film *The Seventh Seal*, referred to in Chapter 2, Death challenges the medieval knight to play chess as a means of postponing the knight's own death. When the game is over, inevitably Death wins and takes the knight's life as the prize. Death is prepared to cheat but always wins in the end. The chess game is a powerful metaphor for millions of different battles with death. Some endeavour to keep death at bay by building up their health, giving up smoking, saying their prayers or making some sacrifice in order to benefit others. Death can be given many names in this active role. It is sometimes thought of as a malign force, associated with such negative names as Satan or the Devil, or with a benevolent God or Allah who nevertheless chooses when each person is to die: 'This night thy soul is required of thee', 'Allah willing'.

Death can also feel as if it is passive. It has been described as a fact rather than as an experience.[1] It just happens, perhaps by chance: why that night for the heart attack, that journey that ended haphazardly in the fatal crash? Death can occur without apparent reason. As the sun rises on the just and the unjust, so also some people live comfortably to an old age, while others die young. The grief felt in the face of the latter is expressed poignantly by William Wordsworth in his long poem *The Excursion*:[2]

> The good die first,
> And they whose hearts are dry as summer dust
> Burn to the socket.

DEATH AND MODERN SOCIETY

People in previous generations were often closer to death than many are today, at least in the so-called developed countries. Advances in environmental health and medicine are increasing life expectancy significantly with all the problems of the human population explosion that are entailed. The time is fast approaching when one in five will be a pensioner and a tenth of the UK population will be over 75 years old.

Nevertheless, death comes in the end and what we think it means is a factor in how we grieve. The impact of belief on bereavement should not, however, be exaggerated. The most optimistic views of a wonderful and certain life to come or a conviction that death is the end for us as individuals is only one element, and the pain of the loss is as real for one person as for the other. Indeed, a sure hope of a life after death can even be counterproductive, if handled insensitively, pushing a person to deny and bury their grief, quite apart from the fear that some people suffer from being judged negatively. In our own time, it is particularly dangerous to make assumptions on what death may mean to anyone, partly because such strong or clear communal beliefs as were formerly more widespread are not to be assumed. Many people work it out for themselves, while others leave a vacuum. If they are not told what to believe, it is as if the question as far as possible is ignored, so that those minds can be concentrated on shorter-term issues of the more immediate moment. Such an approach can work well for many people, but it can also leave them feeling bewildered and unprepared in the face of death. Francois Mitterand, the late French

President, referred to this vacuum when he wrote in a foreword to a fine book about caring for the dying:[3]

> How do we learn to die? We live in a world that panics at this question and turns away. Other civilisations before ours looked squarely at death. They mapped the passage for both the community and the individual. They infused the fulfilment of destiny with a richness of meaning. Never perhaps have our relationships with death been as barren as they are in this modern spiritual desert, in which our rush to a mere existence carries us past all sense of mystery. We do not know that we are parching the essence of life of one of its wellsprings.

The work of the hospice movement, founded in Britain by Dame Cicely Saunders, has been another and significant part of a contemporary response to death. In hospice care, death is respected and the care of the dying considered to be as important as curing other patients for whom there is the possibility of recovery. In the end, of course, there is no cure for that condition everyone experiences: life. At some stage, it is invariably fatal! The evolutionary process depends on life forms that are born, live and die to make space for newcomers, who have the opportunity of being a little different as a consequence. This is both a biological but a personal phenomenon on life's journey. As we grow older, newcomers come into our lives and families, for whom sooner or later we have to make way.

Although we are now repeatedly exposed to images of war and violent death in the media, this may, paradoxically, dull our sensitivity to real death through the distancing effect of film and photograph. Violent death and killing have been prominent themes in entertainment, high and low brow, for a long time. The idea of catharsis suggests that we get rid of troublesome emotions by expressing or experiencing them through drama, art, sport, and so on. Vicariously involved with others, we are plunged into pity, terror or bloodthirstiness, or a combination of all three. Greek tragedy, Roman gladiatorial 'games' and Shakespeare's plays remind us that what is offered through the media is not new. But does repeated exposure to images of violent death help us come to terms with the reality of death? A preoccupation with exciting or tragic images may help us to come to terms with our own fear, while on the other hand sustaining and feeding that fear. Whether or not contemporary dramatics help people come to terms realistically with their own death or of those close to them is another matter. Based on her husband's written account, *Iris* is a study of Iris Murdoch in her declining years with Alzheimer's disease and her husband's efforts to cope, and is one of the exceptional examples of a movie in which dying and death are portrayed realistically.[4]

Most people do not die in battle or a shoot-out, but at home, in hospital or other institutions, from cardiovascular disease, respiratory illness or cancer. When someone does die violently, however, it has a profound impact. Being killed in a crash on the way home from the office on a foggy November evening presents those who mourn with that sense of shock that comes with a sudden and unexpected death.

It was just another Monday morning as the Health Trust human resources department cranked into action. It started as usual with the early regular arrivals making some coffee. They remarked that Jean, one of the longest serving members, had not come in yet. Then Malcolm arrived with the news that she had been killed the previous day in a gliding accident. An empty desk, normally such a mundane phenomenon, became suffused with an aura of sadness. Like a bolt out of the blue, death touched everyone in the department, reminding them of their vulnerability.

DIVERSITY OF BELIEFS

How bereavement works out in practice varies from individual to individual, depending on their personality, life experience and beliefs. The contemporary diversity of belief is not new and is indeed increasing both within society and often within families. This sense of diversity affects us in many aspects of our lives. The songwriter Paul Simon expressed it, for example, when he wrote:

Cultures and artistic movements influence each other by osmosis. The proximity of different cultures, magnified by the speed of technology, offers an irresistible challenge to artists to rearrange languages musically, visually and verbally. Cross-cultural dialogue is inevitable as generations, philosophies and artistic movements bang against each other, intermingle, intermarry and interface. There are many versions of the same truth.[5]

In this chapter, some personal and contemporary ways of looking at the meaning of death are explored.

WHAT HAPPENS WHEN WE DIE?

What happens when we die is for most people a mystery. We do not know, but we have some ideas and perhaps some beliefs and hopes. Often these find expression in reassuring certainties, such as those on a tombstone:

Feare not the grave; assure yourselves
      With Christ your guide to rise,
Who shall prepare your princely seats;
      Your light, your life, your crown
Is he; rewarding all his saints with glory
      And renown.[6]

Another traditional expression of the Christian belief in a personal God and personal survival after death is expressed in the well-known prayer:

We see, to give them back to Thee O God, who gavest them to us. Yet, as thou didst not lose them in giving, so do we not lose them by their return. Not as the world giveth, givest Thou, O Lover of souls. What Thou givest Thou takest not away, for what is Thine is ours also if we are Thine. And life is eternal and love is immortal, and death is only an horizon, and an horizon is nothing save the limit of our sight. Lift us up, strong Son of God, that we may see further; cleanse our eyes that we may see more clearly; draw us closer to Thyself that we may know ourselves to be nearer to our loved ones who are with Thee. And while Thou dost prepare a place for us, prepare us also for that happy place, that where Thou art we may be also for evermore. Amen.

That kind of certainty may have sometimes been as much an expression of hope as faith, a need to believe. The sense that death provided an essential element of justice was also a cornerstone of the efforts in many societies to promote good behaviour. If people seemed to get away with wickedness and crime in this life, their misdemeanours would catch up with them when they died and had to face the ultimate judgement of God, who knew all the evidence. The wool could not be pulled over his eyes by an artful defence! Such faith is still widespread, but it is also being more widely questioned in the modern or post-modern world than in previous centuries.

An example of the varied ways in which belief can be an individual expression, though influenced by a religious affiliation, is a poem by Simon Burne, in which he expresses his belief about death. Though a Christian and a member of the United Reform Church and charity fund-raising director, his poem has echoes of Buddhism in its doubts about the survival of individual, separate consciousness beyond death. The religious content could be seen in his faith that love is ultimate, so central to the Christian tradition. Buddhism, however, also elevates loving kindness as crucial to human development.

When I die I shall cease to be
That flawed clay vessel I once called me.
My spirit like a drop of rain
Will fall back into the sea again.

Once held aloft by the living sun
I fall in peace to the loving one.
Once blasted by the winds above
I merge into the sea of love.

The dirt that made me falls away
To make another me one day.
The joy, the hope, the fear, the pain
Will fill another jar again.

But where I go there is no fear,
And where I rest is very near.
A sea of love where you can swim
And let its healing warmth seep in.

So do not search for me beyond
I'm but one drop in that great pond.
Not lost forevermore but free
Not he nor you nor I but we.[7]

Increasingly the natural sciences are weaving a coherent and unified explanatory web for all phenomena, and many argue that the idea of a soul able to exist independently of the body is more and more incredible. The mystery of death has always taken people to the edge of what can be imagined, and great efforts have been made to find the clues to whether death is the gateway to immortality or extinction.[8] These include trying to make sense of the many descriptions of what have come to be known as 'near-death experiences'. Some of these include the 'great clarity of the patient's consciousness as he looks down on his body from outside, often observing exactly the frenzied efforts of the medical team to revive him'. The accuracy of such reports was striking in that the level of knowledge of what went on would not be normally possessed by the patient, unless he had seen what actually occurred. Nevertheless, such records do not prove to the sceptic that life continues in some way after death. That remains in the field of faith and hope.[9]

Death can be variously seen as helping to give meaning and perspective to our lives. It pushes us to re-evaluate what is really important and to give priority to that. Death is not simply the end of life, but the force that introduces a wholeness and unity into life that is often incomplete until we face our finitude. Some people in their dying have a peace and integrity about them which makes them humbling to be with.[10] They have run their race.

The function of death is to provide the necessary entrance into our innermost selves.[11]

SOME PERSONAL THOUGHTS ABOUT THE MEANING OF DEATH

In the remainder of this chapter, a variety of people in our own time write of their sense of the meaning or meaninglessness of death. The diversity in contemporary culture is reflected in these observations. We can look, for example, in vain for any neat piety from the writer Tim Pears:

Death makes no sense to me. I suppose its meaning can't be separated from the meaning of life. If life does have meaning then it must be part of a continuum, a journey of the soul, in which death, as both alarming prospect and ultimate eventuality, has an equally vital function.

On the other hand life (and death) may have no meaning whatsoever, beyond being part of a chaotic cosmic joke. In which case at least there's a lot of good slapstick, some decent gags, and death makes for a fine punchline.

For those sceptical about survival after death, there is a sense that the person only lives on in memory and can be honoured by the impact they continue to have on those who survive: 'He whom we love and lose is no longer where he was before. He is now wherever we are'. In that way people are remembered through being mentioned casually or formally after their death, often in association with particular achievements to which they have contributed.

Mel Berger, a management consultant, struggling through the impact of the death of his wife, Pam, has written of his thoughts about body and spirit:

> What is death? Why does it happen to people we love, or to anyone? Is it foreordained and written down in an enormous book? Is it simply the result of cause–effect events, for example, by being hit by a car? Or is it a random event like being hit by lightening? There are at least two possible aspects of death, the death of the body and the death of the spirit. The death of the body is more understandable: we can see it, we can observe decay. We can dream of them, we can imagine them walking along the High Street, or even sitting in their favourite chair. We have seen skeletons, and so we can imagine what a dead body looks like. By comparison understanding the spirit is far more difficult to visualise.
>
> If the spirit dies along with the body, we are in a lonely position, especially in an urbanised culture. Life is over and that is that. The person can only live in the memories of others. It is, however, more hopeful to believe that the essence of the person remains, and that it is possible to retain contact in some way. I remember a visit from a beloved cousin in the form of a silhouette against a curtain after he had passed away, only I did not know that he had died at the time of the visit.
>
> If the spirit remains in some way alive, does the spiritual connection remain? If it does, it follows that it will remain with those you love and those you hate: 'I will haunt you for ever' is a threat that signals that the relationship is not over, although you may wish it were.
>
> What does the spirit do all day or however time is conceived on the other side? Perhaps it has its own work to do, past events and people to come to terms with and hopefully to keep a watchful eye towards those left behind and still in grief. Probably over time the need for the supportive contact decreases and people and spirits can get on with doing their own thing. Hopefully in times of need, it is possible to

reconnect with your spiritual partner or friend. Maybe it is possible to reincarnate together in the next life, an exciting and hopeful possibility. But how is the decision taken? And how is it decided where on earth, or not, that the next life is to be lived?

Maybe life and death are like being in a large television with lots of channels, so that we can tune into different people and spirits at different times. Or perhaps the spirit life is more free flowing: no agendas, diaries or appointments on the other side! But at the end I am left with a list of possibilities and questions, but no answers. I am totally baffled and short on faith, which I have heard used to justify too many contradictory beliefs. Instead of the faith that I want, which would feel too much like a highly biased bit of wish fulfilment, I have a void. If the pain of grief keeps going, maybe I will turn to religion or psychotherapy to achieve some healing.

After the catharsis of bereavement, what is left is loneliness, the sense of being alone in the universe. Is that the human condition? Maybe I have reached the point that I need to take more initiatives to refind my connections with people or at least to prop up some hopefully temporary inner subsidence!

Bill Merrington, a Warwickshire vicar, shows how the struggle to make sense of death and dying is not avoided by having a Christian faith:

I think that sometimes that we confuse the issue between after-life and heaven with death. Although death may well be the gateway through which we pass into the other life, it is also a destructive gateway. It (a) is a process of decay, although not spiritually, certainly physically and mentally. How can this be good? (b) It is a severing of relationships, of one's history and sense of belonging on this earth. This too can be painful and damaging. When I therefore see a 97-year-old lady in a nursing home, who may well be looking forward to dying in the sense of entering a peace and an after-life, I am observing the process of death itself that comes through the accumulation of disease and of the destruction of the body. So when people say 'Oh it is release from their illness and pains and weariness', what they are actually saying is that it is a release from their process of death.

We often use the word death in two different ways. At one point we are talking about it being the end, being destructive and of being separated, while at the same time using the word death as a means of escape from these very things into a new life. For those left behind, death in most cases can only be seen in a negative light, which is why we end up with the whole issue of grief. Death brings the severing of affectionate bonds or attachment in the case of children, which inevitably causes a reaction within those who remain. It also brings the recognition that the process of death is in fact taking place within us all. Medicine and science attempt to remove death from our community, but if it is such a good thing, why is it then that we spend millions on attempting to remove it?

Anna Thomas, a primary school teacher and mother, writes from the perspective of one who lost her mother as a young child and then as a young adult both her grandparents, who helped fill that maternal vacuum as she grew up:

> The main thing death means to me is separation. The things that are most important, and what gives me most happiness, are relationships. Death has brought about the end of my relationships with three pivotal people in my life. Because of my religious beliefs, I hope that death is not the end of everything, but it has certainly caused very painful separations.
>
> I hope that death means the gateway onto another plane of existence, but I find the thought of being separated from all who mean most to me unbearable. It feels that it will make any kind of existence meaningless. Life must also be about developing my inner self, or finding out more about it and also my relationship with God, so that I will be better able to cope with separation when the time comes.
>
> My first experience of death was when my mother died. I was too young to understand it or remember, but it has influenced my whole life ever since. I grew up with her absence a daily feature of my life, despite the love I had from my father and grandparents. I looked for her wherever I went, hoping to see her ghost and dreamed of her return frequently. She was spoken about a lot and so I had a clear picture of her, but she was also very mysterious. I felt that I would never match up to her, as death sanctifies people, especially when they die young. So she was to me, as a child, flawless in beauty and intellect and larger than life in strength of personality. She seemed more real and solid than I ever did, until recently. More than 30 years later, I am still experiencing new feelings about her death.

When Kay Walker, a hospice counsellor, reflects on the impact of her father's death. Death itself warrants a capital letter, as if it is a person or a kind of God with whom she is struggling to come to terms. She also expresses that tension that other people sometimes feel between seeing Death as a friend or as an enemy, or even paradoxically both at the same time:

> Death means two things for me – it means people I love leaving me and it means me leaving people I love. The deaths of other people, apart from the people I love and me, is a distant thing but it touches me in the way that John Donne's bell did. It reminds me of losing the people I love – or of them having to lose me.
>
> My work is with people and endings. It has been for some years, both with people who are dying and with those left behind when their loved ones die. I've known in my head and my mind and even a bit in my heart what death is about – but now I've lost one of the most important people in my life, I am coming to know Death with every cell in my body. I am not enjoying it but it is one of the most powerful

experiences I have known. It is like having a child in that way . . . powerful, empowering and wonderful. It's empowering because nothing else matters when you're in the midst of it. It's more painful than childbirth because the pain goes on and on. I know instinctively that I will carry the pain of my father's death in my heart until I die myself.

I don't know if I shall join him when I die. I feel as he did, that I cannot remember anything before I was born and will probably not know anything after I die. So I feel it's best to say all we have to say, do all we have to do and love all we have to love, while we're still alive.

I'm learning that the magical strength I thought I had from him is now in me. A part of me died when he did, but a part of him carries on in me now. I feel good when I recognise some small good thing I do that is like some things he used to do – or even some small not-so-good thing – and I feel proud to be alive, to be like him, and to be me.

My father was cremated after he died. I sprinkled some of his ashes in a river and on the land in an important place for me. I look forward to going back there to visit that river and that land. I hope my children will sprinkle some of my ashes there too.

I'm glad I have lived and am alive. I know I will miss my children and other people I love when it is time to die but I am not afraid of Death. I don't look forward to it – but I think it will be good, like Birth and like Life.

Richard Worsley, a student counsellor, reflects that:

When I am most aware of the immediate, I fear death the least. I have God. I believe in Resurrection. I may be wholly wrong and I face that. If I am wrong, I will meet that (or not!), with equanimity. Yet, I want never to deny the power of the existential angst of death.

Angst, a German word, means the sadness or anxiety that comes with reflecting on the human condition. There is often plenty of angst in contemplating death.

Judyann Roblee, a musician based in Germany, thinks of her struggle with belief and doubt as her ideas change over the years:

I have found that my ideas and thoughts about death have altered and changed shape enormously during my life. I expect that will con-tinue as I get even older. I remember my first thoughts of death as a very small child. At that time it was more of a physical picture in the imagination. Of course, I didn't *think* about it much, and it certainly had nothing to do with me. But the word 'death' conjured up corkscrewing worms turning in the earth. Why worms? I rather enjoyed worms and freshly turned earth. I can still get in touch with this feeling particularly during an aria in Handel's Messiah, where the singer sings 'And worms shall eat your body', with a wonderful 'worming' accompaniment in the orchestra!

I think what I did was more an effort to defend myself from the unknown. If birth was a natural phenomena about which we remembered nothing, death must also be a natural act and somehow we would be prepared and ready for it – as though it would be instinctual. I *still* hope that there might be a feeling of completeness and a readiness to move on at the time of death. But I was disabused of this idea on asking a friend of mine with strong faith dying of cancer if he felt these things.

As I get older life becomes *more* precious each season. At 25 I would have died gratefully, I couldn't bear the thought of being 50 or so. But now I am in my sixties, as I look at the reality of, hopefully, 10 or 20 more seasons, I wish for much longer!

What about the 'life of the world to come'? A phrase we have used all our lives if our lives are lived within the church. This is a hard one to grasp as a real belief for me. What is it? What does it mean? And will I like it? I have had one or two dreams of such strength that I have woken up thinking 'this is what it must be like!' a pouring out of happiness and grief, a release from everything, a joyful peacefulness. I value these dreams tremendously, as being a possible glimpse of the world to come. I wonder too, if there is nothing, a sort of 'lights out' feeling. I fight against this because it seems that I lack faith and perhaps this last leap into the unknown is the greatest leap of faith that we have to take.

From Annie and Titus Mercer, parents and teachers who practice transcendental meditation:

Relief, liberation, adventure, expansion, revelation, new birth, fear of sickness/infirmity/loneliness/leaving loved ones, freedom, reunion with loved ones, into light/infinity/unity/divinity. . . . These words conjure up some of the kaleidoscope of emotions and thoughts associated with death for us.

Coexistence of opposites, that's life (and death).

When individuals try to work out what death means for them, some go on their own journey of exploration into the unknown, often drawing on the ideas, metaphors and myths of their own culture. They may go into poetic orbit with a mystical and exciting belief in the paradox of hope:

Only when you drink from the river of silence
    shall you indeed sing.
And when you have reached the mountain top,
    then you shall begin to climb.
And when the earth shall claim your limbs,
    then shall you truly dance.[12]

But they may also forge ahead with new ideas that may echo other traditions as they go deep into the well of human experience, thought and imagination. Others stick firmly to what they know or believe to be known. For them, any hope of some kind of personal survival beyond death is essentially a human creation, for which there is no evidence. It is a natural expression of the powerful desire and drive to exist, to live and not to come to a full stop.

RITA AND HER GIFT THROUGH DEATH

Death has such different meanings for different people, which, for some, change with their experience of being close to it. That happened to a management consultant and trainer, Jane Trinder, who writes of the life-changing experience for her that came through her colleague Rita's terminal illness and death:

> I had known Rita for a few years as my secretary and then increasingly as a friend. She had won her first battle against cancer a few years previously but was noticing an increasing pain in her thigh. I thought that this might be the cancer returning. This was confirmed months later and Rita decided to retire through sickness to spend more time with her partner. She stayed positive until the end, with her direct sense of humour whenever we saw her.
>
> I supported her by occasional visits and phone calls, but my discomfort of not knowing quite how to help often left me uncomfortable. Rita, however, was always pleased to see any members of the team and keep up with the gossip.
>
> I had not then really come to terms with the death of people I was close to. At this point I thought of death only as a loss and an experience to be dreaded.
>
> However, Rita was to change my views forever and start me on a journey that I had not anticipated. She eventually found herself in a hospice and her partner asked a friend and me to visit. I think in some ways we were both a bit surprised, assuming she would only want those closest around her, and I guess in some ways it stoked our intuition that there was something more to the request. In fact, Rita needed our help in sorting out her affairs, to be able to leave her pension to her partner. As she was gay there was no legal precedent that meant the institution concerned had to do anything. I remember ringing the managing director and asking him to clear the decks, and spent the next 24 hours finding out and clearing through bureaucracy to enable Rita to get her wish. I eventually arrived back in the hospice with Rita and her partner where we had a very private and moving conversation requiring them to document the nature of their relationship. Rita had always been extremely discreet. It was very poignant.
>
> My sense was of being part of a very special moment, which Rita and her partner had asked me to share and felt almost like a marriage ceremony. To see Rita struggling at this point in her illness but so

determined to get the system to work in their favour was a deeply moving experience. It felt that this wasn't just about her but for others who may well find themselves in similar circumstances. Taking my leave of Rita that day I knew would be the last time that I saw her. Before I went to say goodbye, I remember feeling choked with emotion, so pleased to have been able to help but without the words to say anything at all. Rita, however, surprised me as she always did pulling me close to say goodbye and thanks. To this day I cannot find the words to describe what happened in that moment. Her soul seemed to be shining through her eyes and I felt this amazing sense of love and peace, as well as sensing her humour.

Driving home, I found myself starting to compose a poem. Unusual as I have actively avoided reading and writing poems since I was a child. Whole verses flooded my head. Late that night I awoke and went out to look at the stars; my sense was that Rita had just passed away and sure enough her partner called early morning to say that she had died at that moment.

> *Because of You*
>
> I looked into a face of courage
> Both selflessness and selfishness
> To know, and understand, life and death
> To embrace the change of state
>
> I looked into your soul
> And felt the oneness with your spirit
> I glimpsed your journey
> Finding peace in the knowledge you gave
>
> I found that fear is only that
> It holds the space until
> You find a moment of awakening
> Stepping forward not looking back
>
> I can now find my way in the present
> And embrace my future and past
> Giving the gifts that my soul has found
> Sparkling with you in the everlasting light.

In the months following her death, the poem that had flooded my head kept coming into my mind and eventually I wrote it down and took it to a development group I was part of. The facilitator asked me if I would read the poem, which I was very uncomfortable about, but felt that it should be read. The reaction in the room was both very emotional and supportive. The impact of this was to open up a dialogue to share our thoughts and feelings at a deeper level than we were otherwise likely to have reached.

Reflecting recently four years after she died, I realise that Rita gave me a huge gift. Whatever passed between us enriched my life and brought back my creativity and feeling of being part of something so much bigger than myself. My view of death has changed from thinking about endings, to realising that when someone is crossing over it can be a moment of growth and love for everyone. I still feel her presence.

Jane and Rita's relationship illustrates the obvious but sometimes denied or overlooked fact that working relationships can be quite as profound in their own way as relationships outside work. This example also demonstrates how a manager genuinely committed to staff may play a crucial role in something both important and unanticipated not necessarily connected to the job. They may have the ability and perhaps the resource to resolve something that needs sorting more than other friends or relatives of the person who is dying, so long as they do not put up an invisible barrier between work and personal life.

Notes

1 Bayley, J. (1998) *Iris: A Memoir of Iris Murdoch*, London: Duckworth.
2 Wordsworth, W. (1956) The Excursion book 1, line 500, *The Poetical Works of William Wordsworth*, Oxford, Oxford University Press.
3 De Hennezel, M. (1997) *Intimate Death: How the Dying Teach us to Live*, London: Little Brown and Company.
4 Bayley, J. (1998), *ibid.*
5 Simon, P. (1998) 'George on my mind, a tribute to Gershwin on his centenary', *The Observer, Review*, 6 September.
6 Spence, C. (1979) *A Homecoming and the Harvest*, London: Lifestory.
7 Burne, S. (1999) 'When I die I shall cease to be', Rugby: unpublished.
8 Badham, P. and Badham, L. (1982) *Immortality or Extinction?*, London: Macmillan.
9 Sabom, M. (1982) *Recollections of Death*, London: Corgi.
10 The Bishop of St. German's (1998) Speech to the Help the Hospices Conference, London, 17 November.
11 Teilhard de Chardin, P. (1960) *Le Milieu Divin*, London: Collins.
12 Gibran, K. (1926) *The Prophet*, London: Heinemann.

All of the other contributions to this chapter are unpublished notes sent to the author at his request.

Chapter 6

Ignoring death

- The death of death?
- Death happens to other people!
- The death taboo
- A new model of strength
- Unhelpful attitudes towards death

THE DEATH OF DEATH?

Dying is helped by many constructive influences, but the fear of death also tempts people to create a fantasy in which it does not exist: an ideological structure for collective, cultural denial! There are some who even argue that it is unnecessary and avoidable, if only the correct combination of physical and spiritual health is achieved. It is not helped by the Christian idea that Christ has conquered death, as if the kind of death being discussed is the same as the mortality, which is the focus of this book. Even though for many Christians, that notion can be inspiring, reinforcing their belief in a life after death, for others who take it literally and then wonder why they are at a funeral, it is confusing. The problem is that such language is struggling, as death is inclined to do, with ideas that stretch human understanding.

Eternity is 'expressed by the abolition of time as the present participates in the past'.[1] The idea of eternity is that human beings at least can experience and be in, consciously or unconsciously, a dimension that transcends death in the 'eternal now'. Faced with such a notion, many people 'don't get it', while for others it can be accessed, for example, through music, art, nature, meditation or prayer. It is the poetry of mysticism against the prose of materialism. It is in the arena of deeper wisdom or deeper nonsense depending on where you come from.

The literal end of death would be an unmitigated disaster for the human race, as it would presumably not be accompanied by the end of birth, despite current anxieties about reduced sperm counts. Any theoretical commitment to bio-diversity, to sharing our planet with other species, has been drastically sabotaged by the escalating human population explosion that is continuing from the 20th into the present century. There is less and less room for people, let alone other animals and the plants that are needed for food, as greater numbers are squeezed into smaller spaces.

DEATH HAPPENS TO OTHER PEOPLE!

Twenty-first-century western society reinforces the sense that death is something that happens to other people in several ways. Like most people living in the developing world, 19th-century forebears were closer to death as part of ordinary life, as are many people living in other countries in the contemporary world. Advances in environmental health and medicine mean that it will be longer before death makes its claim on most of us. By 2030, there are likely to be twice as many retired people as at the beginning of the century but only about 18% more workers. Instead of having 16 workers theoretically to support each senior citizen, there will be two.[2] The time is fast approaching when one in five living in the UK will be a pensioner and a tenth of our population will be over 75 years old. So many people can live on in old age without the preoccupation with death that was difficult to avoid in the past. When they are younger, an increased life expectancy pushes death down the agenda of preoccupations and concerns. Finally, our sensitivity to death can, as has been discussed earlier in Chapter 5, be paradoxically dulled by repeated exposure through the media to images of war, violent death, dismembered bodies, and so on.

THE DEATH TABOO

The taboo on death involves ignoring or avoiding the subject or talking about it as indirectly as possible. Some of the rituals of death in Britain tend to deny the reality of death. Bodies are removed from hospital wards in trolleys with false bottoms so that people do not realise that a corpse is being carried past them. If a hearse and funeral cortège pass down the street it is no longer customary for pedestrians to stop in respect and solidarity with the mourners. It is often disregarded, with other motorists passing as if it was any other vehicle.

Euphemisms are still commonly used in talking about death: 'he passed on', 'fell asleep' or less respectfully, 'is pushing up the daisies'. The tendency to replace blunt or direct expressions with mild or vague ones can be a form of denial. If you are with someone who is dying or has been bereaved, there is often a dilemma – how to avoid talking about the topic most on both your minds. It can be resolved ahead of time by keeping clear of the person or by making a rapid exit. So the dying and bereaved may notice that they are being avoided by some people and that others are embarrassed in their presence and are clearly relieved to get away from them. By naming death unambiguously it is less easy to avoid its reality.

UNHELPFUL ATTITUDES TOWARDS DEATH

These include:

- death is an evil to be defeated by science or religion, whereas birth is good;
- 'suffering is minimised by avoiding the subject of death'. This attitude is not well founded. Suffering may actually be increased, because the person concerned feels more isolated.
- 'the physical reality of death is more distressing than the imagined reality'. On the contrary, except where there has been serious facial injury, being with the dead body can often be helpful in coming to terms with the reality of death and beginning the healing process of mourning.

Notes

1   Bomford, R. (1999) *The Symmetry of God*, London: Free Association Books.
2   Kotlikoff, L.J. and Burns, S. (2004) *The Coming Generational Storm: What You Need to Know about America's Economic Future*, Boston, MA: MIT Press.

Chapter 7

Preparing for dying and death

It is sometimes said that sudden death is the 'best way to go' but it can be very hard on close family and friends because it gives them no time to prepare. Consider the alternative of a protracted death from the dying person's point of view, however. While it may provide others with the opportunity to prepare themselves for their loss, the dying person encounters what for some can be the hardest of tasks: facing one's own death. Knowing that you are dying, especially if you have not yet come to terms with it, is hard enough. It can be made even harder if those around maintain a conspiracy of silence, so that the dying person feels shut out and even more isolated.

For some, on the other hand, prolonged denial is their preferred way of coping and they do not want to be faced with the truth of their condition. Doctors, nurses, colleagues and relatives have to tread a fine line, picking out the signals of what the dying person really wants to know and talk about. In the past, collusion with denial was the norm, but today more people are saying that to know the truth is what they want in order to base their plans and the strategy of their skirmish with death in reality rather than fantasy.

Patrick, a production manager, was looking more and more ill. He was also untypically for him, asking for time off to see the doctor, but was evasive when asked what the problem was. Eventually, his own manager plucked up some courage and asked him into the office at the end of a day. 'It's obvious that you are not well, Pat, and you may not want whatever the problem is to be talked around the factory, but I would really like to know what is going on. So maybe that way, I can best know how to support you.' To such a direct and perhaps overdue or maybe well-timed approach, Patrick responded openly. He explained that he had lung cancer and that it was inoperable, and in fact he had been told that it might be as short as a few months. His manager assumed that this was the chance for the company to act compassionately and give Patrick time at home on full pay to do what he wanted with his family with whom he was very close and be free from the hassles of work. The offer was turned down flat. Patrick explained that the main reason he had been reticent about his condition, which he had faced up to weeks ago, was his fear that he would not be allowed to continue working.

The manager, in discreet consultation with human resources, agreed to his wishes, but with the proviso that the two of them monitor the situation with weekly meetings. These proved supportive to Patrick and he talked through his ambivalence about giving up work. He liked the job and the people, thriving on the hassles: he'd worked with the company for over 20 years. Stopping work felt as if it would be a death sentence, not an opportunity. But after another two months he did finally accept the offer. Patrick died 10 weeks later. His widow was full of praise for his manager, saying how much the way he had handled the situation had meant to her husband. The manager had treated Patrick with respect, really listened and been person-centred, rather than assuming he knew what was best for him.

Many hope however, that death will occur after a period in which they can manage the end of their life, tying up the loose ends and saying their farewells properly. Some Native American people have a belief that the way a person dies tells the story of how they lived. Dying is a living art, perhaps the beginning of a further passage to something new and unknown.[1]

FACING DEATH TOGETHER OR ALONE

The experience of many who work with the dying is that the latter sometimes know that they are dying even when those closest to them assume the opposite. This assumption may be based on the fact that they have not talked together openly or honestly about death for fear of upsetting each other. Colleagues at work may be the recipients of frankness denied to family members. At times they may help a colleague who has an incurable illness decide to open up to people at home. The sharing of such information between partners, for example, can be not only painful but also deeply enriching to their relationship, as they experience its true quality in the face of perhaps its biggest challenge.

When the dying person knows that he is dying, what is needed is some help to articulate that knowledge. Why should it be so hard to say? Isn't it because everyone else's distress makes it hard to talk, and so the dying person has to protect them? . . . Our experience confirms that the person who says 'I am going to die' does not become the victim of death, but rather the protagonist in his or her own dying. It is a moment of standing up straight again, and of the return of an inner strength that nobody else knew was there.[2]

Even if emotional denial and the stiff upper lip are habitual ways of operating, there is a case for changing the pattern now, because facing death alone can be extremely daunting. To share thoughts and feelings on this issue can bring to the surface the love and commitment, often unspoken, which underpins the relationship. Not to share something as important as the imminent death of a partner can be a tragic epilogue to a relationship; all the more so where the rhetoric of the relationship is honesty and openness.

There are, however, many people who are alone on the road to death. Some patients in hospital have no visitors. Funerals take place with no one in attendance. It is all too easy for people to become isolated in a highly mobile, urban society in which people struggle to discover a sense of community. In many partnerships one person is left who may die alone, especially if an extended family does not exist nearby. In these cases, work colleagues can have a vital role to play in undermining such isolation. Although we cannot share the experience of dying, being with someone as they are dying can feel profoundly supportive, so long as it is not intrusive.

The person who sees death coming has no time to lose. He or she will engage with full force and needs to feel this being reciprocated. I try to make my doubting colleague understand how indispensable the presence of another human being is. There has to be someone else to share this ultimate experience of connection – someone emotionally open, who will not shy away; someone who can remain open to these emotional demands without feeling threatened. This is precisely what those around the dying often find hard to bear, and if they run away so often, it's because they don't understand the meaning of this sudden vitality and they're afraid it can drag them into death as well.[3]

THE TASKS OF PREPARING FOR DEATH

The practical tasks of preparing for death

Death comes sometimes expectedly and sometimes suddenly and out of the blue; so, part of growing up and growing older is to face up to our own mortality realistically. Undertaking the practical tasks is also a means of preparing emotionally, because those tasks involve growing out of denial: 'why bother, it may never happen', even though we know that it will. Of all these tasks, failing to make a will can be the greatest nuisance and (where there are young children) failure to those left behind, but all the tasks warrant attention, if you care for those close to you. Deal with them, the sooner the better: any one of us could be struck down today.

Practical questions in preparing for death

Are you adequately insured?

If you are paying a mortgage, would the outstanding payments be covered in the event of your death? Would your partner, if you have one, have enough to live on if your (separate) accounts were frozen on your death? Does he or she know where this information is to be found?

Have you made a will?

Forms are available from some stationers or newsagents if you want to prepare a simple one and to avoid the expense of going through a solicitor. They must be completed correctly and signed in the presence of witnesses. Have you decided on who you want as executors and asked them if they would be willing to take this on in the event of your passing? Do your close relatives or friends, at least your executors, know where to find the will?

Children under the age of 18

If you have children under the age of 18 and have not specified who you wish to be their legal guardians, the local Department of Social Services in Britain will need to decide who should look after them. If it is not obvious to them who is suitable, they may be put into care.

Have you discussed funeral arrangements?

Sometimes these questions seem too painful to consider and are left to the next-of-kin when the time comes.

In the event of your death, your next-of-kin will need to make these arrangements quickly. Would they know whether you wish to be cremated or buried and what kind of funeral you would want? If you are to be cremated, would you want your ashes to be buried in the crematorium or in another special place? Even if there may be difficulty in burying ashes in various places, there is likely to be little objection to them being scattered discreetly in a beautiful place that is special to you, perhaps on a river, in the countryside or at sea. Is there to be a plaque, sign or perhaps a seat in your memory somewhere, so that those who grieve have somewhere to visit, if they wish?

They may be helped if they know some of your favourite music, songs, hymns or readings that you would like included in the funeral. If they are written down, other people do not have to rely on remembering conversations from the dim and distant past.

Where are your important documents?

Do those close to you know where these documents are, like insurance policies and your will. Are they safe?

What about the practical side of home life?

If only one of a partnership is competent, it may be time for the other one to learn where the stopcock and fuse box are, and to take a turn in defrosting the refrigerator or doing a load of washing.

> Sonia knew that she was terminally ill, and her husband and two teenage children were very dependent on her practically, despite the fact that she held down a demanding job in local government. After she died, they found careful and copious instructions that she had written out for them to follow for cooking, housework and washing. Following those instructions became an important part of them honouring her and learning to live together and to look after each other.

Are there things you need/want to say, practical or emotional, and to whom?

It can be extremely important to some people that the person who has died told them how much they liked or loved them, or what they valued or appreciated about them, and also made it possible in reverse. It may also be very important for the bereaved to know that they have said the same kind of thing to the deceased.

The psychological tasks of preparing for death

Underpinning the practical questions, there are the psychological tasks of preparing for death. At one level, this is a lifetime's work, albeit often at an unconscious level; but if we become aware that our death is getting nearer, it becomes a higher and more urgent priority and nearer the surface of our consciousness. The tasks of preparing for death have been summarised by Sylvia Poss[4] in six parts:

1. to become aware of impending death;
2. to balance hope and fear throughout the crises;
3. to take an active decision to reverse the physical survival processes in order to die;
4. to relinquish responsibility and physical independence;
5. to separate the self from former experiences;
6. to prepare emotionally and spiritually for death.

Not every dying person will need to complete all of these, nor will the process necessarily operate at a conscious level. The tasks involve letting go of this life and, especially in the final two, disengaging from it. At a certain stage, not easy to pinpoint, the dying person may need to stop fighting to get well or even survive. Attachment to and interest in life here and now will consequently weaken. If it is not understood as part of a natural process, this withdrawal from life can feel like rejection and be hurtful to those being left behind.

> Amy had been coping superbly with Jack's long illness, caring for him and keeping the job and home going, until recently when she seemed very moody and depressed. In the office one lunch hour, a colleague asked her how Jack was, commenting that Amy had seemed low lately. Amy described how her husband had always taken such a close interest in the family but latterly seemed to be ceasing to do so. It was as if he was beginning to withdraw from life before he died. To Amy it felt as if he did not love the family or her so much after all. Perhaps he had never loved her through all those years when she had believed that their marriage was just great. But none of this was true. Jack's behaviour was not an expression of how he felt towards the family. His attention was being drawn irrevocably to his departure from this world. In this way the separation that death was to bring was already making its presence felt and Amy was beginning to feel the loss of him.

A great deal of emotional and spiritual energy is required for the work of preparing for death. It is like getting ready for emigration or a world cruise, only more so! The preparation can get in the way of the farewells.

Balancing hope and fear

The focus of hope and fear switches successively from the possibility of recovery, to the quality of life remaining before death, on to the manner of dying and perhaps what happens afterwards. Attention may slide backwards and forwards from one to the other and it is not surprising if perspectives begin to change. When in ordinary life we are hurt or ill, our attention is naturally drawn from where it was to the pain in order to maximise the chances of healing occurring. How much more will this apply when we encounter life's most momentous event?

THE EMOTIONAL RESPONSE TO DYING

A process of mood changes often accompanies the six tasks mentioned above. Though not the same as in bereavement (see Chapter 2), these tasks bear some similarity to that process. In both cases the switch from one state to another may be difficult to predict. But this does not mean that the dying person is going round in emotional circles. The process involves different feelings being dominant at different times. It is as if it is too much to experience them all simultaneously. 'Human kind cannot bear very much reality',[5] at least not all at once.

The emotional stages those who are dying often go through, although not necessarily in the same order, have been summarised in Table 2.[6, 7]

Table 2: The emotional elements involved in facing death

Element	Description
Shock	■ Numbness – protection from emotions, which might otherwise overwhelm
Fear	■ Worse at night ■ Fear of the mode of dying – the need for information ■ Does faith lessen the fear of death?
Acute grief	■ Overwhelming sense of loss ■ Loss of family, friends ■ Hopes for the future ■ Loss of life itself
Denial	■ Healthy defence mechanism ■ Used less as death gets closer ■ Only harmful when blocking the expression of emotional pain
Bargaining	■ Often with God, regardless of faith, or doctors ■ A few more months or a cure in return for altruistic deeds
Depression and sadness	■ The loss of life and relationships and the future, at least in this world
Anger	■ Often directed onto those close at work or home ■ Is it safe to be angry with God? ■ Why me?
Guilt	■ Reviewing life ■ I was so bad that this happened to me ■ Withdrawal, loneliness, regression
Regression	■ Needing to be looked after

Resolution
  Acceptance
  or
	■ Living what life is left to the full
	■ Peaceful detaching and withdrawal from life

Resignation or	■ There is nothing anyone can do about it, so I've got to cope as best I can
Non-resolution	■ Fighting to the very end for survival

No one even hinted to Alan that he was dying even though he was so ill. As a former soccer player on the right side of 40, he could not even wash himself. He seemed to discourage his family from talking realistically and actively planned a trip to Australia to see his brother's family. For his sake, his family in the UK went along with the idea, even though they thought it was totally unrealistic. They assured the hospice staff that he had no notion that he might be terminally ill, and that in their view it was best for him that way. Shortly after his admission, while being bathed by a nurse, Alan started to talk about his condition with insight and knowledge. He cried a lot about the loss of his life and what this would mean for his family. But as he got out of the bath he indicated that he did not want to upset them unduly and started to talk again about the trip to Adelaide.

Denial is a coping mechanism which protects not only the dying person but also other people, sometimes as much or even more. To talk realistically to everyone may be too painful. As time passes, some people want to talk more honestly but find they cannot. Talking can, for some, detoxify their fear. Because of this, a person who appears to be in an extended phase of total denial may respond with great relief and openness to being asked: 'How do you really feel about your illness now?'. Such a question can feel like being granted permission to talk openly.

Someone who is terminally ill may want to protect those close to them from being too upset. They may fear being avoided or shunned, if being with them is too depressing. On the other hand, denial is not just avoiding reality: it can also affirm reality. Being ill and close to death is not the only reality. The reason for not wanting to hasten death is the pleasure and interest that may be experienced about being alive in this world, with all its faults and all the problems of the illness.

There was a lugubrious character in the 1940s British radio comedy ITMA (Its That Man Again),[8] whose catch phrase was 'It's being so cheerful that keeps me going'. The joke was that this was the opposite of what she was really like. Some well-meaning friends, eager not to collude with denial, can be most depressing by homing in on the illness or accident, its treatment (or lack of treatment) and all that is most painful about the situation. They may think that they are sympathising, but are reinforcing a sense of despair and feeling like a victim. It is hard to feel powerful if your physical power is being destroyed. People who in the past have been used to being in charge of their own lives, and maybe those of others too to an extent, regress to a state of dependency. They may be more physically dependent on others than at any time since they were a young child. It is not surprising that they let go of their mental independence at the same time and find all kinds of decisions hard to make, not least if they are struggling with weariness and perhaps pain too. Whereas the person they are visiting may want desperately to get their attention out and onto all kinds of other subjects.

On the other hand, there is the opposite trap of refusing to acknowledge the person's condition and missing or ignoring the verbal or non-verbal signals indicating that the person wanted to talk about their situation and even to be supported in their coming to terms with their mortality. What the dying person needs and deserves from those trying to support them is, if nothing else, the willingness to listen properly, to hear and notice what is being communicated, non-verbally as well as through words, and to pick up and maybe check out the clues and the cues.

Denial provides some temporary protection against the natural emotional pain in most of these stages. It hurts to feel angry or sad or frightened. Most people need to use denial to some degree, especially when the imminence of death has been first acknowledged.

But denial can outlive its usefulness. When it forms a barrier to communication between people who have otherwise had an open and close relationship, it needs to be gently challenged. For others it becomes a firmly held strategy to the end and is best respected.

> I shaved my father with his own razor, slipping glances at his eyes. His pale grey eyes were even paler, farther away. They made me think of Gorky's description of the dying Tolstoy: He listens attentively as though recalling something which he has forgotten, or as for something new and unknown.[9]

SUPPORTING THE DYING

Colleagues and friends will be able to give better support when they know the nature of the main tasks facing the dying person and/or partner. Lacking this knowledge they may find themselves minimising or weakening the available support. For example, they may:

- pretend that nothing out of the ordinary is happening;
- belittle their hope or fear and reinforce the sense that you can feel hope *or* fear, but not both at the same time;
- tell them to keep on fighting when it is no longer appropriate;
- imply that their respect is tied to the dying person's determination, courage and success in looking after himself or herself;
- imply that to let go and even to die might be a kind of failure;
- hint that it was still their responsibility to think about and even take responsibility for their 'dependants' at home or at work;
- disapprove or show embarrassment when the person reflects on death.

Listening can be distorted through all kinds of ideological filters. Sometimes there may be a variation of a religious 'Catch 22'. If your faith is strong enough, you will recover and if you do not, the life after death is better than this one. So you have no excuse for being gloomy. If you are, then you have a problem with your faith: it is just not good enough.

> Alice knew how seriously ill she was. She had given up work and had a bed made up in the living room because she could no longer manage

the stairs. Friends from the church met with her to pray for her recovery, sure that it was God's will that she should get better if only they could all have enough faith. Her husband was not 'religious' but welcomed their support at such a critical time. He encouraged Alice to 'fight' and not give up hope. That seemed essential if she was to have any chance of recovery. Alice did her best, but could sense that her condition was deteriorating; this made her feel more and more inadequate and guilty. Eventually she rebelled and pleaded with them to give her some support so that she could do three things: prepare for death, think about the future of her children after it and begin the heart-breaking task of letting them go. The response of her friends and husband was at first negative. Unaware, they were wrapping in a cloak of piety their inability to face Alice's death. Slowly, Alice helped them gain insight into this so that they could begin to support her in the way that she needed.

The great grief of leaving behind highly dependent young children may be reinforced by guilt. After all, 'being there' is part of good parenting. Sharing some of the pain of that guilt and helping the dying one to think through the best arrangements possible after death may be important ways of supporting someone. On the other hand, if it is too painful to think in detail about the children's future, it may be more important to decide who is to have responsibility subsequently, and then to concentrate on communicating with them and trusting them to do their best.

This can be a crucial part, at the right time, of 'letting go'. Nevertheless, it may be too painful to make a rational decision as to who is to care for the children after a parent dies, and the matter has to be decided by others following her death. This is in part because the decision may depend on some sensitive and detailed consultation with various people, a task that may be beyond the dying person physically and emotionally.

Different questions present themselves in different circumstances. If, for example, the parent that is dying is the main breadwinner, the future financial support of the family may be a crucial element in looking at the potential family and friendship resources needed by the children as they grow up, beyond what insurance cover may provide.

THE HEALING PROCESS

If we are angry, our teeth and fists clench and we want to shout, roar or strike out. If we are frightened, our body may shake, we may sweat. If we are sad, we may weep. In some societies, children and adults are encouraged to express feelings without inhibition. It is assumed that it is natural. 'Better out than in'; 'Better to get it off your chest'.

Unfortunately, our culture has been contaminated by the opposing idea exemplified in the British 'stiff upper lip'. The well-meaning intention behind this is that if someone is demonstrating the physical signs of pain, such as shedding tears, crying out, raging or laughter, which may verge at times on the hysterical, the kindest thing is to stop them. There are two rationalisations at work behind this idea.

First, 'If you can stop the symptoms, you help to stop the pain'. But the opposite is nearer the truth: if you stop the expression of pain, it can become locked in and more difficult to release. Holding back the feelings can cause added stress, whereas to express them can bring a sense of release, which can dissipate tension and help the person relax a little, notwithstanding their situation.

Second, 'It is somehow weak or in the case of men, unmanly, to express strong feelings: weak people are feminine, feelings-dominated and illogical thinkers. The strong masculine person, of either gender, has feelings well in place and can, therefore, think clearly and logically'. This split way of regarding human functioning sees emotion and thought as virtually in opposition to each other, rather than regarding our feelings as part of our intelligence, providing us with valuable information and energy. The emphasis on 'emotional intelligence' aimed at a wider, more balanced approach has, however, sparked its own backlash, in which the fear is expressed that society is in danger of sinking into a sentimental abyss of sloppy thinking with the new respect for emotion.

A NEW MODEL OF STRENGTH

A new model of strength is emerging to replace the image of the brittle, highly controlled man who locks away his feelings through repression and alcohol. In this, acknowledging vulnerability rather than hiding it can demonstrate strength and the release of tension can clear rather than cloud the mind.

The idea that expressing pain somehow makes things worse may have a grain of truth in it. It can certainly be superficially harder for people near them – family, colleagues, friends, clergy, nurses and doctors – who may prefer to pretend that the situation is less upsetting than it really is. It can be uncomfortable, even embarrassing, to be close to someone who is raging or grieving without inhibition. But what this highlights is the need for support for all of the key people near a dying person, rather than a conspiratorial atmosphere of silence and pretence.

There are times when it is appropriate to cover feelings up, perhaps even to disguise them, but there are also times and places to be truthful emotionally with other people. There is a time to weep and a time to laugh, a time for openness and honesty as well as a time for reticence and restraint. Our emotions are no more obsolete than our kidneys or elbows. Whole people with their full potential have and need the capacity to be happy, sad, frightened and angry. They will naturally laugh, cry, rage, tremble, sweat and yawn. Tear ducts have a function for men as much as women, whatever cultural conditioning may say to the contrary.

Emotional intelligence is the ability to use our understanding of emotion in ourselves and others to deal effectively with people, challenges and problems. Emotion is closely related to energy, mood and motivation. Understanding it can help us manage feelings in others and ourselves, so that they can be expressed as well as held back.

People who are dying or bereaved do not need a culture of repression around them at that point in their lives. Happily, there are many parents, teachers and others with responsibility for young people who do not inflict on them such lies as 'big boys don't cry!' or 'showing strong emotion is unbecoming to a woman'. Nevertheless, in too many businesses, 'emotional illiteracy' still continues its insensitive way, creating havoc in the self-respect, morale and motivation of those who feel dismissed and powerless at whatever level or in whatever role. Serious illness or bereavement can reinforce such feelings of inadequacy. On the other hand, the impact of some experiences provide a major learning opportunity that undermines the complacency which so often cloaks emotional illiteracy in an apparently impenetrable cover. The death of someone close for some people creates such an opportunity.

ACTIVE AND PASSIVE RESPONSES TO DYING

Our feelings and values give us the motivation needed to act decisively and with dignity in the face of our own death. Sometimes we need to be highly active in fighting a disease or reaching out in love to someone important to us. Sometimes, however, we may need to be more passive, if the time comes to let go of the struggle to live.

In the range of tasks the dying face, passivity may at times be as crucial and worthy of support as being proactive. A paradox of dying is that the last and hardest demonstration of our maturity may be how well we collaborate in letting go of the independence that we have slowly achieved since our birth. Those who come to accept that they are now as physically dependent on others as they were as a baby may be showing strength no less great for its passivity. It deserves our admiration as much as any more active and obviously heroic feat.

Even more than our encouragement to fight against death, the dying colleague may at some stage need our support in the hard business of letting go of life. We need to be careful in affirming people who are dying for their courage. It can so easily be seen as a coded message to continue to fight death rather than move towards it, let alone perhaps, even regarding it as a strange sort of friend.

Notes

1   De Hennezel, M. (1997) *Intimate Death: How the Dying Teach Us to Live*, London: Little Brown and Company.
2   Charles-Edwards, A. (1983) *The Nursing Care of the Dying Patient*, Beaconsfield: Beaconsfield Publishers.
3   De Hennezel, M. (1997), *ibid*.
4   Poss, S. (1981) *Towards Death with Dignity*, London: George Allen & Unwin.

5   Eliot, T.S. (1944) *Four Quarters*, London: Faber and Faber.
6   Kubler-Ross, E. (1993) *On Death and Dying*, London: Tavistock.
7   Charles-Edwards, A. (1983), *ibid.*
8   ITMA, a BBC 1940s comedy (It's That Man Again) with Tommy Handley.
9   Dodson, J. (1997) *Final Rounds: Father, Son, the Golf Journey of a Lifetime*, London: Arrow Books.

Chapter 8

The practical tasks after someone has died

- Selecting an undertaker or funeral director
- Registering the death
- Funeral arrangements
- Flowers or donations?
- Letting people know
- The will
- Letters of sympathy
- State benefits
- Children
- Throwing things away

The issues considered in this chapter are only relevant to managers, colleagues, human resources staff and shop stewards if the bereaved person is feeling out of their depth, when a diplomatic offer to talk it through may be very welcome. It may be triggered by a helpless or hapless look or something more explicit, such as 'I've never done this before . . .' or 'What the heck are you meant to do now?'. Much of the detail in this situation relates to the British situation, and requirements in other countries need to be checked.

SELECTING AN UNDERTAKER OR FUNERAL DIRECTOR

Be as clear as possible what you want before approaching an undertaker. For example, Nancy and Gordon wanted the body of their young son after his death to stay at home in his room, surrounded by his favourite toys, until the funeral, except for being taken away to be embalmed. They rang several funeral directors in the town, only one of which was prepared to accommodate the wishes of their family on this point. A friend or colleague, on the other hand, on behalf of the next-of-kin, might have done the telephoning and make negotiating on various points, including money, more bearable for them, if they had wished it.

Be careful that in the heightened emotion of immediate bereavement the most expensive coffin and cars to go to the funeral are not chosen inappropriately, unless that is really what is wanted and is affordable. Most undertakers will advise on an inexpensive and simple coffin, possibly even including the biodegradable option of cardboard.

Good funeral directors will concentrate primarily on what are the wishes and needs of the next-of-kin and help to clarify them if they are not sure, while also giving information that is wanted and needed: they will be more marketing than sales orientated. There are still some inadequate under-takers, however, who will be ineffective listeners and regard it as their job to decide what is best, because they are the experts. There is a danger of rushing into decisions at the initial meeting that are later regretted when the bereaved may be still very much overcome by grief. What the funeral director says should be taken into account, and reflected on. Be prepared to tell them you will telephone or contact them in an hour or two, when you have had a chance to think it over.

REGISTERING THE DEATH

Having certified that the person is dead, a doctor gives a death certificate to the next-of-kin or the closest member of the family available. If the person is to be cremated, because there is no way the body can be exhumed if sus-picion arises about the manner of the person's death afterwards, different doctors must sign two certificates. Normally in Britain the death should be registered within five days (or eight in Scotland) with the Registry of Births, Deaths and Marriages.

Whoever goes to the Registry Office needs to take details of the birth-place and date, a note from the doctor and a signed certificate of death. The Registrar provides the certificate for the funeral director that allows the funeral to go ahead. A copy will also be needed to claim any social security money, for which the next-of-kin may be eligible, and, if appropriate, a widow's pension. A third copy may be useful for claiming life insurance payments. So it is often worth getting three or four copies of the certificate for such purposes.

FUNERAL ARRANGEMENTS

These are more fully discussed in Chapter 10, but it is important that the kind of funeral is negotiated that is most appropriate for the person who has died, bearing in mind their wishes and those of the next-of-kin and close family. On the rare occasions when these wishes diverge, discernment, tact and diplomacy are called upon to a great degree, and someone outside the family can help facilitate decision making, be it funeral director, a repre-sentative of a religious or humanist organisation, or even at times a close friend or colleague.

FLOWERS OR DONATIONS?

Some people want to do something tangible and visible of their affection and regard for the deceased. Giving flowers or a wreath is the traditional way of doing this. What to do with any flowers collecting at the church or crematorium needs to be thought about. Often they are just left there, or alternatively they can be taken home or given to a hospital, church or somewhere else where they will be appreciated. Alternatively, an increasingly common choice in the UK is to ask people to contribute to a favourite charity or other cause close to the heart of the person who has died. Once this is decided, it needs to be quickly communicated to and through other people.

LETTING PEOPLE KNOW

To let people know what has happened and is going to happen is a time-consuming task, and while some next-of-kin want to do some, if not all, of it, this is a job that can be undertaken for them, if that is their wish. Care should be taken in reaching precise agreement about the message. Some or all of the following might or might not be included:

- cause, time and place of death?
- was it expected or unexpected?
- how was the deceased before he or she died?
- who are the next-of-kin?
- date, time and place of the funeral, and who is welcome?
- flowers or donation to a charity?
- whether the next-of-kin would welcome contact?

Apart from family and friends, others who may need to be considered might include:

- children's school or college;
- employer, close colleagues, customers and other business contacts;
- trades union and/or professional association;
- the employer of the next-of-kin;
- the deceased's place of worship;
- other organisations with which the deceased was closely involved;
- landlord;
- Department of Social Security;
- executor(s) of the will;
- accountant/solicitor/bank/insurance company;
- provider of any mortgage, loan, hire purchase agreement, credit cards.

THE WILL

If there is no will, an application needs to be made for 'Letters of Administration' from the Probate Registry (or the local Sheriff's Court in Scotland).

LETTERS OF SYMPATHY

Decide whether they are to be answered and whether they are to be kept. It is easy to lose things when in distress. It can be helpful to ask the bereaved person where they would like to keep the letters, and maybe even to help put them there. Later, they can be read through and perhaps acknowledged by a standard card or letter, with some space for a handwritten message, unless the person really wants to answer each one individually. For some, that process can be as much a comfort as a chore.

STATE BENEFITS

If social security grants have been claimed in Britain, it is necessary to visit, write to or telephone the local Department of Social Security office, or it may be possible for someone from the office to call on the next-of-kin. It can be helpful to have someone with you to provide moral support on such a visit. In addition, the local Citizens Advice Bureau (CAB) is a valuable resource for this kind of information. Both addresses are in the telephone book.

CHILDREN

Discuss with children what they want to do, having first explained the situation to them, and support them, whether it is going to see the body, attending the funeral or undertaking a reading at the funeral. Beware of excluding them. They may follow the adult lead or not, but allow them to participate in the grieving. Respect their loss and their need to grieve in their own way and in their own time, but also see Chapter 3.

THROWING THINGS AWAY

It is important that documents or financial records are not thrown away initially, until the financial matters associated with the person's death have all been resolved. Time needs to be taken before unwanted possessions and clothes of the deceased are given or thrown away. This activity needs to be undertaken, but not in a hurry or thoughtlessly, and not necessarily alone. It is an important part of working through the reality of the loss and, for some people, it can be a real help to have someone to provide support. If the next-of-kin is overwhelmed by grief, they may get rid of everything and later regret it. Equally there may be others who are grieving who would treasure something from the deceased if offered in a way that would not be appreciated by a customer in a charity shop.

Chapter 9

Suicide, stress and bullying

- Helping to prevent avoidable suicide
- The impact of suicide on bereavement
- An overview of suicide
- Stress and work
- Bullying at work
- Young people at risk
- Suicide, work, unemployment and men
- Suicide and money
- How can I spot someone at risk of suicide?
- Signs of suicide risk: what can I do?
- Voluntary euthanasia or assisted suicide

HELPING TO PREVENT AVOIDABLE SUICIDE

Suicide can panic people. Those bereaved in a situation where someone has killed themselves need support from people who do not make matters worse by being disapproving or totally horrified by what has happened. Suicide is often, but not necessarily always, a tragic event. If it is not tragic in itself, however, what has led up to it usually is. Work can at times be part of that.

Suicide and some of the ways in which work impacts on it and vice versa are considered in this chapter. Work stress can contribute to suicide attempts, some though not all of which are successful. It can also trigger feelings so desperate that they lead to thoughts of suicide, some though not all of which translate into action. Bullying can be a significant factor in some stress, and so incompetent managers can contribute directly or indirectly to suicides, even if they escape manslaughter charges. A good manager, ensures as far as possible that the right equipment and machinery are in the right place at the right time and well serviced and maintained to do the job. How much more do people need to be cared for rather than wasted as a valuable investment. It is no less the responsibility of the organisation and line manager to ensure that they are in good working order and not liable to break down. Unlike machinery, people have a life, with its hopes, despair and stresses, away from the job, over which the employer has minimum influence. Nevertheless, the responsible manager will:

- be alert to stresses outside of work, which may overload the individual, if pressures are also building up at work at the same time;
- not ignore staff mentioning that they are feeling that they can no longer cope or feel trapped in an impossible situation;
- never ignore people who express thoughts about suicide: allowing them to talk about it never caused a suicide but might have prevented a few;
- beware of and avoid piling up pressure towards breaking point on individuals;
- take account of the different levels of resilience and coping mechanisms among staff;
- respect and take account of their responsibilities to others outside work, especially to children, other dependent relatives and neighbours;
- build a culture in which people are encouraged and affirmed as well as challenged;
- promote a management style in which bullying and harassment are out of order;
- be open to the possibility of careful and informed referral to counselling or other appropriate help, internal or external.

Phil, a personnel manager, had a meeting booked for 2 p.m. with a member of staff and her manager. It was the informal, early stage of a grievance procedure, because the staff member had a number of unresolved complaints. Phil thought that some of the issues were exaggerated moans and groans about the normal ups and downs of work, and he hoped that the meeting would clear the air and put the whole thing to bed. It seemed to work. The issues were got off her chest and the manager, Ian, listened undefensively and promised to sort enough of them out to satisfy the staff member. Meeting over, Phil moved rapidly on to the next item in his diary. That evening he had a long phone call from Ian, who was very low, and had been feeling suicidal. A number of things had been going wrong on his home front, and his self-esteem had taken a battering at work, after some heavy and threatening criticism because a number of his targets had not been met. Being pulled into the grievance procedure, however informally, had felt like the last straw. He finished the conversation by telling Phil that the conversation was off the record and must not go any further.

So Phil had an unexpected sleepless night. The confidentiality had been retrospective, so should he tell Ian's boss? But he knew that his predecessor had the reputation of being a leaky bucket: 'If you want confidentiality to be maintained, the last place to go in this company is personnel'. In the end he asked Ian for a further talk the next day and

shared the issue with him. In that talk, Ian agreed to have some counselling and also to ask for some more time with his manager to review
the targets that he continued to worry about, including the ones that he
felt were unrealistic.

THE IMPACT OF SUICIDE ON BEREAVEMENT

On one level, suicide is another bereavement for those close to the person
and all that applies to bereavement in general is likely to apply to them,
but of course that is not all. When a person who was seriously, perhaps
terminally, ill, takes their own life, it may be experienced, as is usually
the intention, as hastening what might otherwise be a miserable death
rather than as suicide. In cases where death is thought to be suicidal, some
or all of the following *may* apply:

- an overwhelming sense of horror and shock at what the person has
  done and in some cases the manner in which it was done, for example
  shooting, hanging or throwing themselves under a train or off a
  building, adds further trauma;
- guilt and a sense of responsibility for supposedly failing the person in
  some way, for example in not anticipating or sensing what was in their
  mind, in minimising their distress and somehow not making things
  better for them;
- shame that they did not prevent or even worse that they may have, in
  some way albeit indirectly, caused the suicide. This can be particularly
  acute for those with strong religious convictions that suicide is a sin;
- guilt and an element of relief if the person has been abusive/stressful or
  depressing to be with;
- anger that the person has done this, perhaps leaving the bereaved
  person to cope on their own with the trauma, that they have opted out
  by escaping through the gateway of death;
- unresolved or continuing problems, for example financial, perhaps
  caused by gambling, heavy drinking or the use of other drugs, caring
  for disabled or other dependent relatives or problems with parenting,
  can be made worse by the suicide of one partner, leaving the other on
  their own to struggle on.

Many describe the feeling of being tainted by the stigma of suicide. They
feel that others are making all kinds of assumptions about their relationship, condemning them and being wary of them. This can contribute to
a feeling of isolation, especially as most people may think that no one they
know has been close to someone in that situation. For that reason reading
about the experience of other people bereaved by suicide, such as Alison
Wertheimer's book, *A Special Scar*,[1] can be helpful.

AN OVERVIEW OF SUICIDE

Suicide accounts for about a third of the external causes of death in the UK, about 70% more than for road traffic accidents. It has been estimated that about 6,000 people commit suicide annually, an average of one every 90 minutes, and about a further 100,000 attempt to kill themselves, although the rates vary. The level of suicides is not out of kilter with other countries, despite the 16th century French writer Montaigne attributing suicide as the English disease because (according to Madame de Stael) the English were so impetuous and influenced by the opinion of others! The statistics are likely to be an underestimate because the cause of death of a number of people who kill themselves is recorded as something else, either to protect the surviving mourners or because the doctor may not be sure. Arguably in the case of terminal illness, that is the real cause of death even if the actual death has been by suicide.

There are many reasons for taking such a drastic step as to choose to die. Extreme anxiety, shame, depression or physical illness are some of the common triggers: feeling that the future is bleak and without hope. Nevertheless, none of these in themselves explain suicide, because there are others in similar desperate straits who soldier on, sometimes apparently against all the odds. The will to live is deep and powerful, but on the other hand we also have to come to terms with the fact that one way or another we are going to die. Our death is as inevitable and natural as our birth, and so some people begin to think of death as an option in the face of calamity. To seek help to die, voluntary euthanasia, raises further issues, not least because it is illegal in most countries, including the UK. There is a separate section on this at the end of the chapter.

Occasionally someone kills themselves, rather than other people, for a cause: suicide becomes a sacrifice. Others may put themselves in extreme danger, so that they know that they are risking their life. Posthumous Victoria Crosses are sometimes awarded to such men in Britain and the kamikaze pilots of Japan in World War Two were likewise regarded widely as heroes. Unarmed protesters who stood in front of Chinese or Soviet tanks or self-immolating Buddhist monks protesting against the Chinese occupation of Tibet are also examples of the heroism that 'gives its life' for others. Jesus of Nazareth, Gandhi and Martin Luther King are famous examples of people being prepared to offer the supreme sacrifice, knowing that they were putting their life in danger by doing what they believed was right. The west porch of Westminster Abbey in London now has statues in what were empty niches to twelve such 20th-century martyrs from around the world. Suicide bombers of the recent past produce terror and admiration, depending in part on whether you are a target or an ally. Part of the tragedy and the irony is that the cycle of violence of which they are a cog continues after their death among those whose cause they had been fighting for. The fury of those who despise what appears to be indiscriminate targeting is often especially directed at those, often older people who recruit and train them.

In Britain in the past, to take your own life was widely condemned. Until 1961, it was illegal and failed suicides could be charged as soon as they recovered. There was also a widespread belief that suicide was a sin, as well as a crime: the Roman Catholic Church taught that it is a mortal sin, meaning that the person was destined to go more or less straight to hell. The Church of England used to forbid the burial of someone who had committed suicide in hallowed ground. Instead, the body was liable to be buried at a crossroads, with a stake driven 'through the heart' for good measure. The last such burial was recorded in 1823 in London's Hobart Place near Buckingham Palace.[2] Fortunately, in the past 150 years the churches have moved on from such an unforgiving and judgemental attitude so strikingly lacking in the compassion that is meant to be their hallmark. Although the Vatican's 1980 Declaration on Euthanasia observed that suffering has a special place in God's saving plan, few priests today would withhold their pastoral care to someone who took the matter into their own hands.

> The personnel director telephoned the workplace counsellor: 'Do you remember our branch manager, Ian, you saw a couple of years ago? Well, I am afraid he resigned shortly after that, and has had a pretty rough couple of years by all accounts. I have just heard that he committed suicide last week, and I want to offer some sessions with you to his widow, if she wants them. Is that OK with you?' His widow had also worked for the company, but not for the past eight years, while she concentrated on bringing up her three children. The counsellor remembered that he had tried to help with the increasing mess Ian was in, both at home and at work. Before alcohol had befuddled him, he had been a high-flying executive and the company's attitude had been forgiving. They wanted him to sort himself out for their sake as well as his, quite apart from the fact that he had married a delightful and popular member of staff, who was having a very rough time. But it had not worked out. Nevertheless, after the tragedy of Ian's death, the company had been imaginative and concerned enough to offer support to an ex-employee who had left eight years before. Their gesture as much as the counselling, which she accepted, meant a lot to her at a particularly low point in her life.

Suicide is still regarded by some, if not as a crime or mortal sin, then as a sign of mental imbalance. A standard textbook for medical students, published in 1991, observed that 'Suicide is no longer an offence, but properly considered as a manifestation of mental abnormality'. Coroners, recording a suicide verdict, may add while the balance of their mind was disturbed.[3] The assumption is widespread that it is inconceivable that someone thinking rationally could decide to end their own life. Life feels so precious that many people cling on to it at almost any cost. In contrast, the uncertainty of what lies beyond death means, not necessarily with much hope, that many hanker, like Woody Allen, for a return ticket.

In contrast to what many imagine, a study published by the Samaritans[4] shows that a quarter of the population is estimated to have experienced someone close to them dying through suicide. Of these, 11% said the person was a work colleague and 29% a friend, some of whom may have also been a friend at work. In general, suicide rates have been slowly declining in the UK, although in recent years there has been an upsurge in suicide by young men in the 15–24 age bracket, which is 25% higher than the overall figures for men in general.

STRESS AND WORK

The Cost of Stress and Suicide Risk

The changing nature of work has led many people to experience work overload, long working hours, job insecurity and a range of other stress-causing problems in the workplace. This has meant that, over the past few years, many more employees are experiencing higher levels of depression, anxiety and a range of symptoms with which they are unable to cope.

Organisations depend on the existence of healthy staff who are capable of performing their work efficiently. The more successful companies in Britain today pay attention to the health and safety needs of their personnel, recognising that if their structures, policies and working practices reflect the needs of their employees it will increase both quality and output. The Samaritans is the bedrock for all those suffering from stress and depression who need social support and nurture.

Professor Cary Cooper of UMIST[5]

There are some particularly high-risk occupations. Indicators of this include high stress, isolation and access to resources that make it physically easier to commit suicide. The importance of the latter has been highlighted by the apparent link between the number of suicides among men in particular and the catalytic converter, which became mandatory for all new cars in Britain in 1992. In the following four years, deaths by car exhaust poisoning (classified as poisoning by other gases and vapours) dropped among men by a recorded 37%. The President of the Royal College of Psychiatrists at the time, Dr. Robert Kendall, observed that the introduction of catalytic converters had decreased the number of suicides without substitution of other methods.[6]

The suicide risk among male farmers decreased over the 10 years 1982–92 but remained high, accounting for 1% of all male suicides during that period. Farmers and their wives averaged one a week. The availability of firearms may have been an exacerbating factor, with 38% of male farmers using this method compared to 5% of all male suicides. The wives also used firearms in 10% of their efforts to kill themselves as opposed to 1% of all

Table 3 High-Risk Occupational Groups in England and Wales

Occupational group	PMR* suicide risk (%)	Number of suicides 1988–92
Men aged 16–64		
Vets	361	18
Pharmacists	199	18
Dental practitioners	194	18
Chemical scientists/engineers	156	38
Forestry workers	155	27
University academic staff	152	27
Farmers	145	177
Medical practitioners	144	60
Women aged 16–59		
Ambulance women	402	3
Vets	387	3
Government inspectors	365	3
Medical practitioners	322	25
Nurses	154	247
Pharmacists	141	4
Literary/artistic professions	112	42

Note
* PMR is the Proportional Mortality Rate, a measure of suicide risk. The average for men aged 16–64 and for women aged 16–59 = 100. Thus a PMR of 365 for female government inspectors indicates that this group is at 3.65 times the risk of suicide as the average woman between aged 16–59.[7]

female suicides. Farming remains a potentially lonely occupation for those who do not immerse themselves in the community in other ways. In Britain, it has been subjected to a series of continuing crises associated with supermarket tactics, government policy, so-called 'free trade', globalisation, genetic modification, the side effects of chemicals, foot and mouth and other diseases. Tasks previously undertaken by many people working on the land have been mechanised. If organic farming grows in popularity, more people will be involved in it, because it is more labour intensive than most other modern farming. As a consequence, farmers will again stop being quite so isolated, quite apart from the environmental and human health benefits.

The availability of the means to commit suicide is also illustrated among those who take their own lives in the health care professions, choosing self-poisoning to a larger degree than in the population as a whole. Nurses, for example, accounted for 5% of all female suicides during the years 1982–92.

People undergoing difficulties in their lives outside work are vulnerable to being steered towards suicide by insensitive managerial behaviour.

George had taught at a leading secondary school for 15 years, but his teaching had become an increasing struggle over the past year. During that time he had had two major operations, despite which he was in almost continuous pain. At the inquest, his widow said: 'He had no doubt that he would continue, until he was summoned to a meeting in which he was given an ultimatum. He had three weeks to improve his teaching, which he had not previously been made aware of, otherwise he would be required to leave. He came out of that meeting feeling his integrity, which was unquestionable, had been questioned and he felt undermined and humiliated'. A few days later he killed himself, having written two notes, one to the school chaplain and the other to the headteacher. The school declined to comment at the inquest.

Suicide can also be triggered by a potentially lethal combination of organisational change combined with what is sometimes called 'macho management'. Typically, the latter is a form of bullying in which a manager abuses the power that he has to threaten and intimidate his staff without concern for the pressures they may be under at or indeed outside work. One such example came with the threat of redundancy.

A large company was going through some radical change, involving a plan to 'down size' or reduce staff numbers by nearly 50%. One of the managers, Tom, had witnessed a new senior manager, who knew none of his people, come in and deliver a threatening pep talk. In this he promised that at least half of them would be gone by the end of the year and it was up to them to demonstrate that they were worth keeping and better than the others. This was in a culture that had previously been characterised by teamwork and a pride in pulling together. Shortly after that talk, one of Tom's long-standing engineers, Ryan, excellent at his work but not overly self-confident, disappeared. It was Tom who, after a 24-hour search, found Ryan's body. It was in his car, on one of the more distant of their scattered sites: Ryan had shot himself through the head. Tom who knew and liked him had never witnessed a sight as distressing before in his life. The tragedy was traumatic for Tom on many levels. Fortunately, he had some debriefing in the psychology department of the local hospital at the firm and insistent instigation of an enlightened trades union official, who became involved. Tom's own line manager had not recommended that he have any support, and appeared to be oblivious to the possible need for it. To rub salt into an already very raw wound, his main concern was that Tom keeps the matter away from the media.

There was widespread concern by Tom and some of his fellow managers that a number of newly appointed senior managers were adopting a macho style incompatible with the values and approach to managing change, which had underpinned what the company was officially and publicly advocating.

This was one of a number of incidents that reinforced the concern that such a style can put some insecure staff, with significant financial responsibilities, under the kind of unnecessary added stress, which may be the thin edge of the suicide wedge. The irony was that the company subsequently put a high priority on helping redundant staff find a new direction and path in their lives.

BULLYING AT WORK

Bullying, harassment or ridicule occurs at work, sometimes to the point where for a particularly vulnerable person with low self-esteem, it can become unbearable. There is inevitably a fine line between firm management and bullying, but that distinction is being increasingly recognised and acknowledged.[8, 9, 10]

Bullying comes in many shapes and sizes, but may include:

- public humiliation;
- constant negative criticism without any balancing encouragement or respect;
- shouting, sarcasm or sneering;
- threats of discipline, dismissal or demotion;
- unrealistic deadlines, doomed to failure;
- vague, incompetent, unclear instructions;
- lack of regard for the person's life outside work;
- arbitrary refusal for leave, time off, going home on time;
- diminishing the person or their job;
- consistently dismissing their ideas and suggestions;
- blocking promotion or training opportunities;
- negative appraisals;
- sexist, racist, ageist or homophobic behaviour;
- sneering at or attacking the person's religious, political or other beliefs or values;
- sneering at or mocking the person's appearance, accent or family;
- physical intimidation.[11]

The fear of being accused of bullying makes some managers feel that they are themselves victims, which of course they can be. Some manipulative staff become sophisticated at threatening managers with the bully label if disciplinary action is taken against them. Where disciplinary action is needed, however, competent managers in a competent company will take it with care but without fear or favour.

YOUNG PEOPLE AT RISK

Suicide accounts for 20% of all deaths among young people and is the second most common cause of death among young men, claiming more lives than cancer.

Research summarised in a 1997 Samaritans report[12] indicated that the rate of suicide attempts by young men had doubled in 10 years, although subsequently it appeared to level off, but is still much higher than it used to be. Work, unemployment and study issues were contributing factors nearly twice as often with that age group as among all adults attempting suicide. A total of 56% of young men who had attempted suicide had such problems. They were only exceeded as a possible trigger by relationship problems with a partner or another family member. Work, unemployment and study issues were way ahead of such difficulties as those concerning friendships, money, housing, alcohol, drugs, social isolation or psychiatric illness.

Bullying can impact particularly hard on younger people, and they are especially at risk to it. Such behaviour is disproportionately targeted at younger and newer employees. Some older people, whose coping strategies have been developed over time, may cope more effectively with it. At a younger age, some of those same people may not have built the necessary confidence, perspective and skills to contain, combat or in some way deal with bullying. Consequently, it can be magnified to the point where some young people, especially, come to believe that the only option left is to kill themselves. Among this age group, the quality of the parental relationship is an important factor: research indicates that young suicide 'attempters' report less perceived support and understanding than other adolescents who are depressed.[13] The support of even good parents can seem extremely remote to a young person at work, especially if they have gone away from home, as for example in the armed services.

For such youngsters, a good manager, team leader or supervisor may have some of the characteristics of a good parent, an adult role model, who is perceived to be on their side, firm but fair but also, above everything else, encouraging when self-confidence and esteem are shaky. The same effect can come through a good teacher, although large class sizes make that difficult, whereas a reasonably sized span of control at work makes a human and humane working relationship possible, if the culture reinforces it. In addition, reviving apprentice schemes or developing mentoring for young employees are additional ways of reducing the risk of depression or despair getting out of hand for this age group.

All of this should alert responsible organisations, military or civilian, to ensure that young people are managed properly. The spotlight needs to be particularly vigilantly directed against induction procedures and the early days of employing or training young people so that humiliating, embarrassing or degrading rituals, which still unofficially linger on in some organisations to their shame, can be rooted out. They put those in their care unnecessarily at risk and promote a culture of disrespect for others. The macho rationales used in their defence should be treated with the contempt that they deserve, but more than that. Those involved in such rituals need to go back to first base and be helped to understand that they are wrong and indeed a warped route to promoting resilience and toughness. There are much more emotionally literate ways of doing that.

SUICIDE, WORK, UNEMPLOYMENT AND MEN

In a study on trends in suicide and unemployment in Scotland 1976–86, a period during which there was a national increase in suicides among men of 50%, an association between the two was found among men nationally, though not among women.[14] Because this was not consistent regionally, a rise in unemployment may not be a direct cause of the large rises in suicide rates. Unemployment can be isolating, especially when individuals are picked off, but it can also be a cause of solidarity with others. As redundancy becomes more common, the stigma may lessen, especially for those who find new employment or start on a self-employment route relatively quickly. Nevertheless, the financial pressures on families associated with unemployment can create a bitter cocktail of anxiety, guilt and anger among many people, not least those for whom self-esteem is tied into their success as breadwinner.

Unemployment among older people can cut both ways. For some it is not so bad. Their children, if they had any, are beginning hopefully to be self-supporting and the mortgage, if there is one, is paid off. The redundancy or early retirement package can mean that the financial pressures are not too onerous. So it is often an opportunity to do something different after years struggling with the daily or nightly round of toil. For others, whose self-esteem and social contact were tied up with their job, its status and trappings, the experience can be devastating. The relative lack of money may make it worse, because the financial needs of an expensive family may still be considerable or because their life-style was inexorably tied into conspicuous consumption. The need for another comparable job may feel urgent, and being apparently too old to be employed embittering. The scrap heap is a common metaphor for an unhappy middle age, let alone old age, for too many in a society obsessed by youth without a balancing regard for the wisdom of experience and 'the elders'. Companies that arrange effective outplacement for those who are made redundant are doubly wise. This process both minimises the risk to those made redundant as well as following the common-sense principle that 'the beginning of motivating those who stay is how you treat those who go'. To make people redundant and ignore the responsibility of providing support to them to cope with the experience and to shape up to the next stage of their life is deeply irresponsible.

In general, men are more at risk than women (75% of suicides are by men), although there is a marked and worrying exception among young women between the ages of 15 and 19.

SUICIDE AND MONEY

The funeral is often delayed after a suicide by the inquest that is required in England and Wales. A slightly different procedure is followed in Scotland. Life insurance policies frequently include one-year suicide exclusion clauses. The intention behind this is to discourage people with large debts seeing life insurance and suicide as a way of sorting out a family financial crisis. Insurance companies vary as to how rigidly they interpret such a clause. Some consider each case individually, and may use their discretion to pay out after they are satisfied that they have established all the relevant facts. Pensions are not usually affected by suicide, although some pension plans with integral life insurance may also include a suicide exclusion clause.[15]

The following two notes sections may help people to spot someone at risk of suicide and also to think about what to do in those circumstances, and are notes from the Samaritans, reproduced here with their permission.

HOW CAN I SPOT SOMEONE AT RISK OF SUICIDE?

Use what you know

Has the person you're worried about experienced any of the following:

- recent loss (a loved one, pet, job);
- the recent break-up of a close relationship;
- a major disappointment (failed exams, missed job promotion);
- a change in circumstances (retirement, redundancy, children leaving home);
- physical/mental illness.

Has he/she:

- made a previous suicide attempt;
- a history of suicide in the family;
- begun tidying up their affairs (making a will, taking out insurance);

Visual clues

Is he/she:

- withdrawn;
- low-spirited;
- finding it difficult to relate to others;
- taking less care of themselves;
- different in some ways, for example unusually cheerful;
- tearful, or trying hard not to cry;
- more irritable;
- finding it hard to concentrate;
- less energetic, and seems particularly tired;
- eating less (or more) than usual.

Things to listen for

Does he/she talk about:

- feeling suicidal (it's a myth that people who talk about it don't do it);
- seeing no hope in the future, no hope in life;
- feeling worthless, a failure;
- feeling very isolated and alone;

- sleeping badly, especially waking early;
- losing their appetite or eating more than usual.

The Samaritans, telephone: 0345 90 90 90

Source: the Samaritans

SIGNS OF SUICIDE RISK: WHAT CAN I DO?

Trust your instinct – if you're concerned, you're probably right. Ask how the person is feeling and listen to the answer. It's difficult to support anyone who is suicidal on your own: encourage anyone feeling low to seek emotional support, from family, friends, medical services, the Samaritans and others.

Ring the Samaritans yourself on 0345 90 90 90. We may be able to contact the person you are worried about.

Source: the Samaritans

As far as the last point is concerned, talking a concern over with either an experienced colleague, counsellor or the Samaritans may help you decide both what to do and, as important, how to do it.

If you suspect someone with whom you are working is feeling so low that they are contemplating suicide, should you mention it? Norman Keir, a former chairman of the Samaritans has written:[16]

> A common reason for not enquiring about suicidal feelings is the fear that to do so with someone who may be at risk could be dangerous. This is quite unfounded. Taking one's life is hardly an option one would adopt because someone had put the idea into one's head. Indeed a working party of the Royal College of General Practitioners advised that 'there should never be any hesitation in asking a depressed or agitated patient if he has wanted to kill himself'.

Keir emphasises the fundamental importance of listening, which should underpin everything that is done in the name of the care of the suicidal. 'On the face of it, the process of listening might seem superficial and trivial, whereas when undertaken correctly, it is one of the most potent techniques in resolving suicidal crises'.

VOLUNTARY EUTHANASIA OR ASSISTED SUICIDE

Someone who is close to someone who is dying sometimes finds them both struggling with the feeling that the person who is ill wants to have some control over the timing and manner of their dying. This may seem like one of the few remaining things that they want from life, and they also may feel very frightened of the implications of not having that sort of power. Euthanasia can then cease to be a theoretical subject for a debate but a desperately urgent and personal matter. The principles of active listening, in which judgement is suspended, become the more important in such a situation rather than offering premature advice or an outline of one's own views on the subject. This section has been written especially for the manager or colleague who has not given much thought to this issue, and needs to think it through a little in order not to panic and to give effective support to someone struggling with it.

The debate about voluntary euthanasia continues, even while it is illegal in most countries. To seek help, especially that of a doctor, to hasten death is based on the sense that people should have a 'right to die' or rather have 'individual control, as far as is possible, of the process of dying'.[17] One study suggested that as many as a quarter of the 3,696 people interviewed would prefer the option of an earlier death in certain cases, rising to 35% in those over 85, so the issue is of concern to large numbers of people in one way or another:

- 28% of respondents and 24% of the deceased had expressed a view that an earlier death would have been preferable.
- 35% of the over 85s, compared to 20% of younger people, said that they wished they had died earlier.
- Only 3.6% of those who had died were said to have asked for euthanasia.
- Religious faith, social class and place of residence had little bearing on people's views about euthanasia.
- People who had experienced hospice care were, if anything, more likely than others to express the view that it would have been better to have died earlier.
- Fear of becoming dependent was a greater factor than pain among those expressing these wishes, although cancer patients were more likely to be motivated by the fear of pain.

Euthanasia is seen by its advocates as a means of securing the option of a gentle, dignified and timely death for those otherwise condemned to die long after an acceptable quality of life has ceased.

The opposition to euthanasia is based primarily on some combination of three arguments. The first is that it is unnecessary, the second that it is open to serious abuse and the third that it is morally wrong. There have been great advances in pain relief and control in medicine, although the standard of knowledge in this area is more reliably and consistently spread within the hospices and among specialist doctors and nurses, including Macmillan nurses, than among doctors and hospitals in general. Enlightened and skilful doctors will not 'officiously strive' to keep a patient alive, irrespective of the quality of life or the pain that the patient may be in. Many general practitioners admit to using opiates to relieve pain, which may shorten life. Nevertheless, even in hospices, there may be patients who desire to end it all, but who are unable to do so. One condition that has evoked such a desire among some patients is motor-neurone disease.

Advances in medicine, especially in the field of pain control, have been used to argue that euthanasia is not needed in the world of today.

> Martin was an engineer in a large food production company. His young wife, Rosemary, had suffered from a debilitating and terminal form of cancer for six years, and had reached the point where there was no more treatment available at a time before the hospice movement had got going in his part of the country. For some time, Rosemary, knowing that her death was getting nearer, had indicated that she wanted to die in her own home, and not go back into hospital. Her doctor, on being pressed by her, had acknowledged that after chemotherapy and radiotherapy and several operations, they had reached the point where no more active treatment was possible. At that time, barbiturates were commonly prescribed as sleeping tablets and Rosemary had collected a supply over the months. One night she had a recurrence of severe pain, which would have meant that she would need to be readmitted to hospital. So she asked for her husband's agreement that she should take the tablets. They had discussed this option thoroughly before several times. Rosemary wanted to have some control over her own death and had decided that she had been into hospital enough times. Not wanting her to suffer any more, Martin agreed and a little later held the tablets for her while she held a glass of water from which she sipped and took them one by one, before falling into a coma. She died peacefully without regaining consciousness.
>
> Martin's grieving was complicated by the knowledge that, even though he believed that he had done what was right by Rosemary, if the way she had died had become public knowledge, he might be prosecuted for manslaughter. He was fortunate in that he was able to share the truth of her death in confidence and without guilt with a counsellor with whom an enlightened manager put him into contact. Keeping such a secret would have increased the level of stress that had built up during his wife's illness and after her death. This was caused by trying to support Rosemary, to ensure that their young children were adequately cared for when she was in hospital, as well as after her death, and to maintain his effectiveness at work over an extended period.

The fear of abuse in voluntary euthanasia is both political and personal. In Europe, the Nazis, under Adolf Hitler, pursued murder under the guise of involuntary euthanasia as an instrument of policy towards Jews and other groups of people, until their military defeat in 1945. The more personal fear is that ruthless relatives, after the money of a sick person, may prevail upon them to opt for euthanasia. Alternatively, a sick, disabled or elderly person may choose it because they do not want to be a trouble or in the way of other people.

The moral argument is similar to that which used to be deployed so widely against suicide. Life is sacred. We have no right to determine when a person dies: 'thou shalt not kill'. It has been pointed out, however, that what this Commandment in the Book of Exodus, chapter 14, delivered via Moses, meant was that a Jew must not murder a Jew, but that when it came to dealing with their enemies, different criteria applied. The Egyptians found this to their cost when they tried chasing the people of Israel through the Red Sea.

In addition to the Netherlands, another modern government has tried to thread its way through this tangle by giving circumscribed rights for voluntary euthanasia to the terminally ill. The Rights of the Terminally Ill Act came into effect in Australia's Northern Territory in July 1996:[18]

Rights of the Terminally Ill Act 1995

Legislative Assembly of the Northern Territory

- The Act confirms the right of a terminally ill person to request assistance from a medically qualified person to voluntarily terminate his or her life in a humane manner.
- The patient must be over 18 and terminally ill.
- Assistance may be by administering appropriate drugs or supplying them for the patient to self-administer.
- The illness must be causing severe pain/suffering.
- The patient must not be suffering from treatable depression (an independent psychologist must confirm this).
- The doctor must share the same first language as the patient or have an accredited translator present.
- The patient must be offered and must positively refuse all further palliative care.
- There must be a period for reflection between the first discussions and the final decision.
- The doctor must be present until the patient has died.
- Insurance will not be affected.
- Foreigners will not be able to travel to Australia to benefit by the Act. [Immigration laws bar visitors in poor health.]

A 1999 court ruling in Britain found a general practitioner not guilty of murder after he had admitted to prescribing opiates to a terminally ill patient in order that suffering be relieved in a quantity that he knew would also bring about death.

In a Dutch study[19] of 'different exits', the majority of deaths are those where no end-of-life decisions were made: people just died, but the authors identified five other categories. Two were familiar: nearly 20% died from administering pain-killers in large doses and about the same proportion of people died from the decision to forgo treatment. In most of these cases, doctors estimated that life had been shortened by less than a week, with patients hopefully being spared a week of misery. The other three categories were for voluntary euthanasia (about 2%), with rather less for doctor-assisted suicide and the alarming category of the intentional ending of life without the patient's request: 'It could have taken another week before she died. I just needed the bed'.

In a 1997 Leader,[20] *The Economist* observed that: 'It would take an extraordinary law that could disentangle, in every case, the motives of mercy from those of easy disposal'. Nevertheless, the Leader concluded that it would be an abdication of moral duty if human beings did not at least make the attempt to produce such a law. Before embracing such a law, however, doctors and politicians should consider other ways to shore up the dignity and self-determination of the individual. The Leader provided a useful checklist of what most of us would want for each other, whether as colleagues, friends or family:

- patients should be fully informed about what is being done to them;
- patients should receive the best care possible, including palliative treatment, that is often scandalously neglected;
- patients should be able to determine where they die, at home, in a hospice or in hospital;
- patients should have the right to refuse medical treatment, either at the time or through advance directives such as Living Wills.

A Living Will or Advance Directive[21] is a form expressing the individual's wish to their doctor but does not ask the doctor to do anything against the law. It usually asks that the following applies if the person suffers from one of a list of conditions and becomes unable to participate effectively in decisions about their medical care:

- In the event of two independent physicians (one a consultant) being of the opinion that there is no reasonable prospect of recovery from serious illness or impairment involving severe distress or incapacity for rational existence:
  - ❑ that I am not subjected to any medical intervention or treatment aimed at prolonging or sustaining my life;
  - ❑ that any distressing symptoms (including any caused by lack of food or fluid) are to be fully controlled by appropriate analgesic or other treatment, even though that treatment may shorten my life.

The debate will continue as people consider living wills and talk among themselves and with their doctors. Whether (and if so how) a doctor should help a patient to let go of life remains a private matter between the two of them and, perhaps, their next-of-kin, within the boundaries set by the law and personal and professional ethics.

Notes

1 Wertheimer, A. (1991) *A Special Scar: The Experience of People Bereaved by Suicide*, London: Routledge.
2 Davies, J. (1997) *Choice in Dying: The Facts About Voluntary Euthanasia*, (forward by Dirk Bogarde), London: Ward Lock.
3 Davies, J. (1997), *ibid.*
4 The Samaritans (1996) *The Cost of Stress*, Slough: The Samaritans.
5 The Samaritans (1996), *ibid.*
6 Laurance, J. (1998) Why suicide rates in men are dropping, *The Independent*, November.
7 The Samaritans (1996), *ibid.* Source of table: Kelly, S., Charlton, J. and Jenkins, R. (1995) *Suicide deaths in England and Wales 1982–92: the contribution of occupation and geography*. Population Trends 80.
8 Keir, N. (1995) 'Suicide and counselling', *Insight*, no. 3, March.
9 Ryan, K. and Oestreich, D.K. (1991) *Driving Fear Out Of The Workplace*, San Francisco, CA: Jossey-Bass Publishers.
10 Adams, A. (1992) *Bullying at Work*, London: Virago.
11 Adams, A. (1992), *ibid.*
12 The Samaritans (1997) *Exploring the Taboo: Attitudes of Young People Towards Suicide and Depression*, Slough: The Samaritans.
13 The Samaritans (1997), *ibid.*
14 Crombie, I.K. (1989) 'Trends in suicide and unemployment in Scotland 1976–86', *British Medical Journal*, vol 298.
15 The Samaritans (1997), *ibid.*
16 Keir, N. (1995), *ibid.*
17 Welsby, K. (1996) Survivor's lament, *Independent on Sunday*, 30 June.
18 Davies, J. (1997), *ibid.*
19 Welsby, K. (1996), *ibid.*
20 *The Economist* (1997) 'The right to choose to die', Leading Article *The Economist*, 21 June.
21 The Voluntary Euthanasia Society *The Advance Directive*, London: The Voluntary Euthanasia Society. www.ves.org.uk and www.livingwill.org.uk

The community, death and bereavement

Chapter 10

Funerals and rites of passage

- Support over the funeral from the organisation
- The purposes of the rites of passage
- Cremation or burial?
- Offering the body for medical education or research
- Cremation
- Greener funerals
- Funeral costs
- The funeral
- A Service or Meeting of Thanksgiving or Remembrance

Funerals are, for many, essential as the collective goodbye and tribute and expression of love and affection for the person who has died. Others regard them as a trial to be endured. They are strange affairs too, inspiring all kinds of responses. Tennessee Williams puts into the mouth of Blanche in his play *A Streetcar Named Desire* describing the impact on her of the funerals of her culture: 'And funerals are pretty compared to deaths. Funerals are quiet, but deaths – not always. Sometimes their breathing is hoarse and sometimes it rattles, and sometimes they even cry out to you, "Don't let me go!" Even the old sometimes say, "Don't let me go!" As if you were able to stop them! But funerals are quiet, with pretty flowers. And, oh, what pretty boxes they pack them in!'.[1]

SUPPORT OVER THE FUNERAL FROM THE ORGANISATION

'A Checklist for Possible Support over the Funeral from the Organisation', is included in the checklist section at the back of the book. The various decisions about the funeral are often resolved within the family. Other next-of-kin appear to know exactly what they want without much support from anyone in particular. This chapter is not included to encourage people at work to interfere needlessly; but there are circumstances where the issues considered here impinge on the workplace. In some situations, the dying person or the next-of-kin, may feel uncertain about what to do about 'rites of passage'. Especially if the death is unexpected, those tasks can be an added source of stress.

So, some bereaved people may panic and feel overwhelmed by the burden of feeling that they do not know what to do and where to start. Not all funeral directors, ministers of religion or others who might lead funerals are sensitive and helpful. They may pressurise the next-of-kin towards their preferred way of doing things, which may or may not be appropriate or what is really wanted. Some next-of-kin value being told what the drill is and fitting in with the traditions to which they have allegiance. On the other hand, the next-of-kin end up feeling thoroughly disempowered, when they need to feel the opposite. Someone at work may pick up signs of this and support them diplomatically to make their own way through this maze.

In many cases, colleagues will of course themselves have a personal relationship and friendship with the partner or child who has died, especially where the gap between work and home is not too rigidly defined. There is often a difference between work located in cities and those in smaller towns or villages. People commute, for example, from far and wide to central London jobs, making it less likely that they would see colleagues outside work.

Where there has been a death in service, the employer in consultation with the next-of-kin may undertake the organisation of a 'rite of passage'. Examples of this include the armed forces, police, fire and ambulance services and the churches. Tact and sensitivity are important so that the next-of-kin do not feel sidelined or flattened by the company. In this chapter, the aim is to help such a person decide what to do (or to help their manager or other member of the organisation guide them towards appropriate decisions).

A rite of passage often takes place in a different place to the funeral, where the person who died has strong associations. The funeral of John Smith, a former British Labour Party leader, was in his native Scotland, on Iona, while his Service of Thanksgiving took place in London in Westminster Abbey, across the road from where his work was based. After a colleague, Tony Milne died in 1994, a firmly non-religious Memorial Gathering in Celebration of his Life was organised at a club in London, whereas his funeral had been some time before where he had lived in Kent.

THE PURPOSES OF THE RITES OF PASSAGE

Katherine Ashenburg has spoken of the changes over the 20th century in western attitudes to grieving:

> There's no need for a leave-taking ceremony or a funeral, but just about every culture in the world seems to have one. There's no need to wash

a body. Why do it if you're going to burn it or put it in the ground? Yet so many cultures do it.

After World War I, the sheer volume of losses was overwhelming. By 1917, people in England stopped wearing black because every family was in mourning, and it was undermining morale. When the only child of Sir William Osler [a prominent Canadian-born physician] was killed in 1917, they just filled the boy's room with flowers. There was no ceremony.

The 20th century way in the West is to mourn in our hearts. We're praised for doing well and almost acting as if nothing has happened – going back to work and wearing red, or going to the movies and things like that. . . . It seems that from 1920 to 1990, the pendulum had swung so far from the full-blown mourning of the 19th century that mourning became socially unacceptable. I think the pendulum is beginning to swing back.

When the war ended, people never wanted to see mourning clothes again. Plus, modernity was dawning in the sense of hope against child-hood illnesses. There was a feeling like we've conquered death, which of course we haven't.[2]

The phrase 'rite of passage' is used to describe rituals that take place after someone has died. The 'passage' can be thought of as the deceased person's passage from this life into their future existence or their existence in eternity, if it exists, or for those left behind from life with to life without that person. These rites play an important part in our collective as well as individual coping with death. Although there are many variations, the themes of 'rites of passage' in different cultures tend towards meeting five basic needs to:

1   Do something appropriate with the dead body relatively quickly before decomposition makes it an added source of distress and offence.
2   Say farewell to the person, at least in their existence in this life, whether or not their death is regarded as the end; and perhaps also to help the dead person's spirit on to the next phase of their existence.
3   Honour and celebrate the person who has died.
4   Acknowledge and begin to come to terms with the reality of the death.
5   Provide a focal point for collective grieving and comfort for supporting those people who are grieving the most.

The rites of passage commonly used in Europe come in various combinations. They are discussed below, but in summary are:

■   a Service of Thanksgiving or a non-religious Thanksgiving Meeting or Gathering, which may be held at the funeral or some time after it. In the past, this event tended to be called a Memorial Service.
■   a funeral at which the body is present in a coffin, not necessarily in a place of worship. Such services in some Christian traditions maybe in the form of a Requiem Mass or Communion service.

- the farewell to the body, often with a short service and commendation, at a crematorium, or by the graveside after the funeral.
- In the case of cremation, the ashes may be subsequently buried or scattered either in the crematorium or in a specially chosen place.

A variation on these is to hold a short funeral service for just a few of the closest relatives, and possibly friends, to say farewell to the person and for the disposal of the body. A Service or Meeting of Thanksgiving, an event in which the person and their life can be celebrated by a much wider and larger gathering, can follow this private service straight away, the next day or rather later.

In the case of cremation, this is sometimes planned the other way round. The funeral director takes the coffin with the body away straight after the main service or meeting so that everyone can go to the wake together. The cremation takes place privately, with or without a few close mourners, later that day or shortly afterwards. This is especially worth considering if the main event is some distance from the crematorium.

The social get-together afterwards is as important in its own way as the funeral and complements it. The mourners can talk and reminisce about the deceased and reconnect with each other. It can be based in the home or a more neutral setting, such as a pub, community or church hall or a hotel. A possible disadvantage of the home is the pressure on those most affected to stay until the end, rather than have a place to which they can retreat, if they feel the need. On the other hand, it can be comforting to have people there.

CREMATION OR BURIAL?

The next decision to take is what combination of rites of passage to have. The person might have decided this before they died or it has to be quickly resolved by the next-of-kin when the time comes after the person has died – or is just about to die.

Twentieth century population growth and technology contribute indirectly to the unfamiliarity of death. A funeral used to be held in a local church, in the churchyard of which the body would then be buried. People went to the same place for rituals surrounding birth, marriage and death. Thus, symbolically in the midst of life we encounter death and vice versa. And since, for many, the church was part of weekly, if not daily, life, it was easier to sense, with William Blake, that:

Joy and Woe are woven fine,
A clothing for the soule divine.
Under every grief and pine
Runs a joy with silken twine.[3]

When the churchyards started to fill up, cremation became a solution to overcrowding, especially in densely populated urban areas, although it was illegal in the Britain until the end of the 19th century. The Cremation Society was formed in England in 1885 and the last opposition to cremations was removed in 1964 with the lifting of the Vatican's ban on the practice. It is now in Britain the main way of disposing of a body, with an estimated 71% of funerals involving it; although this figure is proportionately lower in Scotland than in the more crowded countries of England and Wales.[4] While there may be much to recommend cremation, it led to the development of places associated only with death. In crematoria, death is separated from the rest of life – an unconscious and unintended expression of our contemporary enthusiasm for specialisation.

Behaviour is strongly influenced by culture. In the multi-cultural society of early 21st-century Britain we are beginning to realise that other traditions have helpful ways of responding to death that do not minimise it. Cultures are never static and there are signs that the British one is becoming more open and flexible. There is a more widespread sense than there used to be that people need to do it 'their way' and be respected for doing so. Notes on some of the beliefs and customs around death of some of the main religious and irreligious traditions in Britain form part of the next chapter, 11.

When a member of staff dies, whether they were still working or retired, colleagues who knew them are usually very welcome at the rites of passage. By going, the dead person is being honoured and their family supported. Sometimes several colleagues going, especially if the person has worked for a long time for the same organisation, can be especially valued. The weight of numbers of people coming to a funeral is often noticed and a source of comfort to the close family. It is as if the regard for the person who has died is being affirmed by the numbers of people from the community, including the workplace, who give up their time to come. A book or card, which those attending sign, can reinforce that afterwards, as the next-of-kin may be hardly aware of who else was there.

Letters and donations to a nominated charity (or flowers) can reinforce that same message. Among the colleagues may be the line manager and/or the most senior director or executive in the organisation who knew the person who has died. Their attendance can have a powerful representative role, particularly if the senior person has a deserved reputation for behaving with integrity and for being caring.

In the same way, a representative or two from the company can also be supportive to a staff member at a rite of passage for one of their particularly close relatives, such as a partner, parent or child.

Often the members of staff will organise the event without needing help from their workplace and will indicate one way or another whether work colleagues are welcome. There are times when this is not the case if the boss or company, through the stress it put the staff member under, is thought to have contributed to a premature death. If in doubt, give permission and encouragement to others close to the person to attend.

OFFERING THE BODY FOR MEDICAL EDUCATION OR RESEARCH

The first decision to make is what to do with the body. An interim possibility, before cremation or burial, is to offer the body or part of it for medical education or research or for transplant surgery.

A body can be offered in the will or by the next-of-kin after someone has died to be used in the training of doctors or more rarely for medical research. Generally, badly diseased bodies will not be suitable, so be prepared for the offer to be turned down for this or some other reason. If the body is accepted, the remains will normally be returned, perhaps a year later, for disposal. This needs to be prepared and planned for, so that the next-of-kin is given good support, whatever the decision, and decisions about rites adjusted accordingly.

CREMATION

If the body is to be cremated, the question follows: what to do with the ashes? Arrangements can be made for them to be buried in a crematorium garden, churchyard or scattered in a chosen place. Ashes are biodegradable and soon absorbed into land or sea. They can be scattered or buried straight into the earth or buried in an urn, or container, which will – at least for a time – stop them from intermingling back into the earth.

There are four options for the crematorium chapel. The first is to ask someone to take the service, such as your local minister, priest, rabbi or a friend. The second, is for it to be taken by the local member of the clergy who may be on duty that day. The third is to ask someone from an organisation such as the British Humanist Association to lead a 'non-religious' service or meeting. The fourth is for friends or relatives chosen by the next-of-kin to lead the service. Lastly, there is the choice of no service at all. One problem with a crematorium-only funeral is that the time is usually severely restricted and it can be hard to avoid it feeling hurried or perfunctory. On the other hand, that time is fine for some people. The minimal option is a cremation. The service will often be restricted to 20 minutes or so, unless a double slot is booked beforehand.

Crematorium chapels are restricted in space and often smaller than most churches. In a well-attended funeral, some of the congregation, unable to get in, might be gathered around the door straining to hear. If that is anticipated, it should be possible to organise audiovisual equipment for outside. An example of this on a very large scale was the broadcast from Westminster Abbey of Diana Princess of Wales's funeral to the crowds outside, many of whom joined in the hymns and prayers as well as applauding her brother's powerful address. The ashes are usually available later the same day or the following day to be buried or scattered, an event in which close family can participate, although they need not do so.

GREENER FUNERALS

Increasingly, a green approach to death is raising questions about the burning of coffins. Alternative approaches are being developed. These, for example, include the burning of the body in a body bag allowing the coffin to be passed on or otherwise reused or the use of cheap, biodegradable coffins made from cardboard or other material.

For the environmentally conscious, burials are sometimes now taking place in woods with a commemorative tree planted over the burial place. The Bishop of Coventry, for example, consecrated a woodland burial site for such a purpose in Coventry in 1995. The wood is not just a place of death, but a living and beautiful place. The tree represents new life coming from the old, a symbolism equally accessible to someone who is agnostic or religious.

FUNERAL COSTS

There may be scope for assistance with funeral expenses from the employer, especially if the person has been killed in action or at work, though as in most issues around death and bereavement, great sensitivity is needed in thinking through the implications and in broaching the subject with the next-of-kin.

Funerals are not cheap and in the UK over £1,000 is usual, whereas across the English Channel the cost can be rather less. Depending on inflation, for example, a British funeral director may charge about £800 for providing a relatively cheap wooden coffin, caring for the body until the funeral and a hearse (the specially adapted large car) to take the coffin to the funeral. Hardwood coffins are much more expensive in financial as well as environmental terms. The hire of extra cars to carry mourners might be a further £80 each, church and clergy £80, although an organist and peal of bells could double that. Doctors' fees for cremation certificates and the fee to the crematorium could run up another £300.

THE FUNERAL

A minister of religion often leads a funeral: for example, Anglican clergy conduct an estimated 70% of funerals in England. The Anglican Church's General Synod has discussed the degree of preparation and support given to the bereaved through these processes. Sometimes this is exemplary with sensitive pastoral care and a service that honours the person who has died. Sadly some funerals in crematoria can appear to be impersonal and even peremptory. Some clergy may be well meaning but can be crassly insensitive. 'The vicar stood to make a sermon. The exposition was lengthy . . . We were told how Jesus was our friend, and why Christianity was different from all other religions, being more than a set of rules. There was no reference to the life we were celebrating, or even to the reason why we were there . . . As the sermon took its course, the temperature in the congregation seemed to drop by about 10 degrees'.[5]

While the idea of a painless funeral may be over optimistic, a well-prepared and sensitively conducted funeral can and often does bring great comfort, even though it may have been dreaded in anticipation. The ceremony needs to be well done in order that the person to whom people are bidding farewell is honoured through it.

Because work is such a significant part of the lives and identity of many people, it often features prominently one way or another in a funeral. This may include someone from work speaking about the person. The former England and Surrey cricketer Alec Stewart's experience of the difficulty of doing this for his team-mate Ben Hollioake, after his fatal car crash, is far from unique:

> I was asked by his family to speak at his funeral and it was the hardest thing I have ever had to do. My subject was Ben the cricketer and friend. The most difficult part was trying not to break down and somehow, my voice faltering, I got there. I'd taken my example from Adam [Ben's brother] when he'd spoken the previous afternoon at the service. He's one of the toughest guys I've ever met, yet even he broke down, as you'd expect after such a tragedy. How he got through that I'll never know. It was very moving and touching and we all cried our eyes out those two days: a tragic loss to a wonderful family and his many friends.[6]

Cricketers playing at that level have to be tough as well as skilful, called upon to face a very hard ball bowled at them at times very fast: 100 miles an hour has been clocked. Stewart rates the different kind of toughness we need to face in death as greater. His way of describing the tears the Surrey players shed also exemplifies the emotional literacy that is becoming more widespread, epitomised by the slogan 'Big Boys Do Cry', which neatly contradicts the opposite that was so widespread a generation or so ago.

In death, we are all equal in the sight of God or, if there is no God, at least in the eyes of enlightened men and women. There is a widespread sense in both humanism and in many religions that a person, despite all our limitations and foibles, is very special in him- or herself, irrespective of fame, success or tribe. It is character and personality that makes anyone unique, and that is what needs to be honoured in a funeral. This was well expressed in the funeral of a good friend, Tom Kinsey, in the poem:

> Not how did he die, but how did he live?
> Not what did he gain, but what did he give?
> These are the units to measure the worth
> Of a man as a man, regardless of birth.
> Not what was his church, nor what was his creed?
> But had he befriended those really in need?
> Was he ever ready with word of good cheer,

To bring back a smile and to banish a tear?
Not what did the words in the obituary column say,
But who was sorry when he passed away.[7]

To ensure that it is neither rushed nor overcrowded, a service or meeting needs to be planned to include as many as want to come, for a reasonable length of time, say between 40 to 60 minutes. For cremation, the short service can be held first or the next day in the crematorium, if it is some distance from the church, mosque, synagogue, temple or meeting place, so that the service in the latter can be held immediately before the wake. This logistically may be the only way of allowing the mourners to meet socially together after the funeral, which is an important part of the whole process.

We live in a period of unprecedented diversity in what people believe or do not believe, and in religious and non-religious allegiances. People are encouraged to work out their own values and beliefs rather than take them from the dominant belief system in their culture, whether religious or atheist. This means that there are also correspondingly more choices about where to hold a funeral, who to involve and what to include.

George, a computer programmer, died young and his widow wanted a service for him that honoured who he was. He was an agnostic Stoic, with a deep love of music. She was a Roman Catholic and they also had many Jewish friends. The funeral was planned to reflect both his scepticism and also the beliefs implicit in the other two traditions among his family and friends so that they could all feel that the service was one in which they could genuinely be part of. It took place in the local Roman Catholic Church, whose priest cooperated fully in supporting the people who took part, including a Church of England minister. Prayers were prayed to God rather than through Jesus, and it was noted that the Lord's Prayer of Jesus was originally a Jewish as well as subsequently a 'Christian' prayer. It was suggested that the word, God, be given a personal meaning by each individual, as the focal point of what they most honour – whether it is the Creator of the Universe, the Holy Spirit, goodness-truth-and-beauty or the love and justice that exists among people at their best. A musical improvisation by a double bass-playing, sailing friend of George was an especially moving tribute transcending verbal language, which can so easily tie us up in conflicting knots.

Expressing and valuing such diversity of belief as a healthy reality can dispel a sense of hypocrisy and bring people together in unity, which is particularly important at a funeral.

This sense of not so much burying our differences as living in peace together in a period of grieving is sometimes experienced in public as well as private life. When prominent politicians die, the tributes paid to them by opponents, as well as allies, are very different in tone from the adversarial insults so often traded in the House of Commons. In the face of death, disagreements, squabbles and conflict can often seem petty and differences, which can inspire such passion on other days, trivial.

Some people plan their own funeral down to the last detail and find comfort in doing so. It reduces the decisions that the next-of-kin has to make. Others neither want nor feel able to do this while they are alive, but may tell a close friend or family member a few items they would like included. The person closest to them may make notes of favourite poems, music, readings or hymns, leaving them to make the actual arrangements after the person has died. As noted above, some clergy, like funeral directors, are more open to suggestions than others.

To what extent should the service be taken 'off the shelf' rather than being developed by those close to the deceased? A balance needs to be struck, depending on the wishes of the deceased and next-of-kin. For many, a familiar, well-tried liturgy is right, but even then there will be a chance to choose music or hymns. For others, much more input to both the shape and content of the service is wanted. Such a wish to be involved will hopefully be welcomed but may be resisted: there are still clergy who expect to have the final say on every detail, but they are a decreasing minority. Most people taking funerals, including representatives of the British Humanist Association, will welcome suggestions for music, prayers, readings and offers of help to play or speak, so that the service really reflects the person who has died. Some eyebrows were raised at the funeral of a friend, which began on his instructions with: 'There's no business like show business'. It set the tone for a service, which was authentic and moving, evoking laughter as well as tears, which was of course his intention all along.

When my father died, we had to cope with an undertaker who was not a skilled listener and tried to tell him and his family what was proper. It turned out to be something of a struggle, not the best time to have to negotiate hard. Nevertheless, we ended up getting most of what the family wanted. This included my father's embalmed body staying in his home for six days until the funeral, allowing members of the extended family to make their own farewells in their own time and in their own way. Then the evening before the funeral, his body in its coffin was taken to the church. It remained there overnight, with members of the family taking turns to keep vigil with it.

When my mother died, on the other hand, a very different funeral director concentrated on understanding and implementing the wishes of the family. So when we wanted four members of the family to carry her coffin into and out of the church, he readily agreed – only asking to meet them briefly to instruct them on the best way to lift, carry and lower the coffin, so that no mishap occurred. We were very conscious after my father's death that it was only our confidence and toughness that enabled us to get our way and how easy it would be for people feeling much more shaky to just give way. On the other hand, such a directive approach from a funeral director would be reassuring for some people wanting to let the expert take over at such a difficult time.

A SERVICE OR MEETING OF THANKSGIVING OR REMEMBERANCE

A Service of Thanksgiving to celebrate the life of the person as well as mourn their passing, separately from and after the funeral, takes place for a minority of people but it can also be helpful. Until relatively recently, the phrase Memorial Service was common, although it was a 20th century phenomenon, with the Memorial Service for Queen Victoria marking the beginning of what soon came to be a tradition for the famous or publicly distinguished. A Requiem Mass honours the person too but its purpose is also to pray for their soul in its onward journey through purgatory and, hopefully, to be with God.

At the beginning of the 21st century the Memorial Service has been largely replaced by the idea of a Service or Meeting of Thanksgiving. The positive element in this is the celebration of a person's life, with grief implied but largely under the surface. It can even reflect denial in the bereavement process if the funeral occurs soon after the person has died, when grief is raw, even if mixed with shock and denial. The service needs, however, to avoid the tyranny of the positive in which pretence and the stiff upper lip rule supreme. That balance is captured by C.S. Lewis when he wrote that 'the pain now is part of the happiness then'.[8] There usually needs to be some acknowledgement in both the funeral and Thanksgiving of loss and sadness, perhaps reflecting to an extent the movement through some of the worst and most acute grief.

Such a service can be like a marker of the end of the period of formal mourning, even though that may not be either intended or expressed in most British cultures. Memory in the ritual of memorial can recall all that was good and loveable about the person, which is the raw material of why their loss is the subject of sadness. At its worst to deny sadness might re-inforce the isolation of those people who cannot escape from their grief amidst a crowd of people who appear not to really care that much.

Whether it's a Meeting or a Service depends on what auspices it comes under. Humanists and those who do not think of themselves as religious may plump for a Meeting in a secular setting. Quakers also use the term Meeting, while a Service implies a religious dimension, albeit in a gathering of diverse views and beliefs, the common currency of contemporary society.

Notes

1   Williams, T. (1984) *A Streetcar Named Desire*, London: Methuen.
2   Brady, D. (2003) 'Mourning in America: an interview with Katherine Ashenburg', *BusinessWeek*, 23 October.
3   Keynes, G. (1962) *The Complete Writings of William Blake*, London: The Nonesuch Press.
4   Christian, K. (1997) *Handbook of Religious Trends 1998/9*, Carlisle: Paternoster Publishing: 47.
5   Blacker, T. (1998) 'The spirituality of sad old hippies', *The Independent*, 15 December.

6   Stewart, A. (2003) *Playing For Keeps*, London: BBC Books.
7   Anon.
8   Lewis, C.S. (1961) *A Grief Observed*, London: Faber & Faber.

Chapter 11

Culture, religion and death

THE INFLUENCES OF CULTURE ON OUR RESPONSE TO DEATH

This chapter, for some, will need an explanation, as many people find the words spiritual, religious and transpersonal meaningless, resonating neither in their experience nor their outlook, even though culture may be a concept with which they are more comfortable. After all, western societies are often now called secular, which is contrasted with the religious or sacred, but they are also characterised as diverse, in which people have a wide variety of religious and irreligious convictions. For many people, what they regard as spiritual or religious is very important to them. Equally, others may think of themselves as Christian, Hindu or Muslim but are relatively indifferent about how that compares to the business of getting practically on with life in the short term. A number of people in England and Wales were asked, for example, whether 'religion was important to them' in the 2001 Home Office Citizenship Survey, published in May 2004. Whereas fewer than 10% of agnostics and atheists not surprisingly answered negatively, those who self-described as Christian only hit 15–25%, depending on their age. For Sikhs, Hindus and Muslims, the percentage rose to 50–75%, with the highest figures for the latter two among the youngest age group surveyed, 16- to 24-year-olds.

If colleagues are to be well supported, we need to be sensitive to all of this. Where belief is important to the bereaved person, it should not be blanked out, perhaps especially if it is very different to our own. It may also be useful to have some idea about their religion's (or humanism's) line on death and bereavement, including the question of rituals.

As we become more aware of our diversity, so we also can come to realise some perhaps unexpectedly common strands within that diversity. Katherine Ashenburg has explored this in writing of her daughter's bereavement after her fiancé had been killed in a car crash. 'When I saw Hannah, who has no interest in history, doing things that other cultures had institutionalised as part of their mourning, I thought there might be something more universal and more profound about these things. She had time lines for moving her engagement ring from her left hand to her right hand. She wouldn't socialise in groups of more than two or three. I later learned that that's a rule of Orthodox Judaism, that you're not allowed to be in large groups for a year after a serious death.'[1]

Human history has often involved societies in which the dominant belief systems, political and religious, have been defined by those with the most power and been imposed, sometimes brutally, on the rest. In some parts of the world, the past couple of hundred years have seen massive change for at least three reasons. They can be summarised as, firstly, the rise of democracy as an idea and a system; secondly, the realisation, through science, philosophy, theology and linguistics, that religions and the way people think are evolving and subject to change; and thirdly, travel, migration and communication have increased the experience and knowledge of different cultures and belief systems.

In contemporary multicultural society, as people take seriously the variety of religions in the world, working out what they really believe can become part of their spiritual journey. Thinking for myself has always been part of what produces diversity in the first place. So individuals throughout history, endeavouring to love truth or God 'with all their mind', as Jesus suggested to his followers, have found themselves questioning and challenging the dominant position taken within their country or society. This questioning has led to the formation of splinter or separate religious groups. Thus, Sikhism grew out of Hinduism, Lutheranism out of the Catholic Church of Rome, whereas atheist Stalinism was a reaction against what was taken to be the superstitions of Orthodox Christianity in Czarist Russia.

Today, people feel freer than their forebears to think 'the unthinkable' and to express beliefs without fear of persecution. Glen Hoddle, however, might not agree with that after being sacked as England football manager in 1999, apparently in part for expressing a politically incorrect version of his faith in an interview with a journalist. Further confusion was caused because Hoddle is a Christian who apparently believes in a form of reincarnation. Faith or faithless labels are commonly used to describe packages of ideas and practices to which you are expected to assent if you own them. Hindus, Buddhists and others, especially if their religion originated in Asia, can believe in reincarnation, but not Christians, Jews or Muslims. For them, it's the life after death, but not in this universe, or nothing.

Belief, however, has a personal as well as a communal meaning. As individuals think and meditate about the mystery of life and death, and open themselves to different experiences, thinkers and ideas, we may as individuals end up believing all kind of things. During our life journey, our beliefs may change over time, without them necessarily jumping religious ship and disowning our main religious or irreligious allegiance. On the other hand, there are many who get on with other aspects of their lives, without particularly bothering about religious issues. They are content to allow their religion or irreligion to provide them with a set of beliefs, which they accept and which resolves some of the uncertainty of 'not knowing what to believe'. Such a view may be linked to a respect for authority or the experts, who are taken to know more about a particular subject than we do, because they specialise in it.

Religions have developed with many strikingly common themes. With their ceremonies and mythology, they are superficially so different that it has been easy to exaggerate their deeper differences, especially if politically they were being used as a mask for competition and military conquest. The multicultural diversity of belief permeating more and more countries in our global village presents us with both an opportunity and a challenge. The opportunity is to discover what is good, interesting and inspiring in the beliefs of others and to outgrow tribal exclusiveness on the religious (or atheistic) front so that we make peace. The overwhelming challenge is to allow this process to grow on the basis of global justice, sensitivity and mutual respect, in which the gap between rich and poor does not continue to grow at the expense of the latter and the environment.

In the workplace, all of this applies in different ways. Instead of a taboo on talking religion and irreligion, we need to develop ways of learning about the beliefs and practices of others in a way that enhances mutual understanding instead of antagonism and suspicion. The basic communication and listening skills needed at work are all that is required for this to take place, alongside the core conditions of helping listed in Appendix 2.

Religions and non-religious philosophical systems, like atheism, humanism and stoicism serve to provide a common language and way of making sense (or nonsense depending on your perspective) of existence. They can help us, individually and collectively, to develop a moral basis and a sense of purpose for our lives. Their language at its most powerful is poetry, mythology, music, art and architecture, rather than prose. All of these contribute raw material for the rituals surrounding dying and death and our attempts to communicate about and make sense of them.

Humanism can help us look at death thoughtfully and maturely, as, for example, when the Roman emperor, Marcus Aurelius (121–180 AD), wrote:

> A little while and you will be nobody and nowhere, nor will anything which you now behold exist, nor one of those who are now alive.

> Nature's law is that all things change and turn, and pass away, so that in due order different things may come to be.[2]

Religion can provide a sense of perspective, which is not always that different, such as the biblical invocation from the Book of Ecclesiastes, chapter 3, verses 1–4:

> For everything its season,
> and for every activity under heaven its time:
> a time to be born and a time to die;
> a time to plant and a time to uproot;
> a time to kill and a time to heal;
> a time to pull down and a time to build up;
> a time to weep and a time to laugh;
> a time for mourning and a time for dancing.

Or religion can express the need for hope within despair and poverty, as in the Christian Aid prayer:

> Though what is past
> may be full of loss
> and the present insecure,
> never shall despair
> take away our future.
> Give us the seeds of hope, O God,
> and we will clear the ground,
> plant and weed, and work and laugh,
> our harvest safe in your hands.

SPIRITUAL SUPPORT

Spirituality is an elusive concept but can be thought of as the mix of attitudes, beliefs, feelings and practices beyond the rational and material, which are nevertheless important to the individual in providing 'an ultimate sense of meaning and purpose'.[3] Such a definition goes wider than religion, which is one but not the only channel through which spirituality can be experienced. Some atheists, for example, think of themselves as spiritual. The transpersonal is a term not used much outside counselling and psychotherapy, but means that which is beyond time and space, the profound experience of being at one with humanity, but without any necessary dogmatic trappings.

Intolerance sabotages empathy. Some religious people can be derisory of atheists and humanists, but it can also work the other way round, not least among some in the helping professions. The spiritual, religious and transpersonal can all be dismissed as nonsense, though not necessarily all by the same people. Bernard Moss has argued that 'religious and spiritual matters were not only debunked in such circles – they were regarded as being fundamentally suspect, the smoke screen left by primitive superstition, which needed to be blown away in order to establish social work on a sound value base'.[4] He quoted Lloyd, who observed that 'one legacy of social work's embracing of Freudian theory in the late 1950s and 1960s has been a continuing mistrust of religion and a tendency to dismiss by association the significance of spirituality'.[5]

Moss concludes that 'the experience of loss has a profoundly spiritual dimension to it'. 'Spirituality is something we all share and, if professional workers deny this for themselves, they are likely to deny it for the people whom they seek to help.'

The sense that our consciousness has a spiritual dimension, which permeates and perhaps also transcends our physical, emotional and mental experience, can also be thought of as the root of 'authentic religion'.[6] When death causes a sense of the spiritual to rise to the surface of our awareness, it can become a necessary ingredient in the wider support that may be valued. So whether or not we think of ourselves as 'spiritual', supporting those for whom it is important requires us to treat the concept with interest and respect as we focus on their inner as well as their outer world.

Ritual provides a social structure for support and mourning in which the place of the spiritual is central. To express its meaning is elusive and difficult, which is why some religious writing can feel lifeless and empty and why music, art and poetry are more likely to hit the spot.

Spiritual support can also be important on a one-to-one basis. A shared silence is often an important way of being with someone near the end of their life or recently bereaved. Either way, it gives them a chance to go deep into the reality of what is happening while having the reassurance of another human being close by in case the experience is too overwhelming. Ministers of religion are not the only people able to offer prayer for someone who is dying or bereaved. It can mean a great deal to share a prayer or meditation. It requires the courage to offer something in a relaxed and natural way while having the restraint not to press it or spin it out unduly. On the other hand, if the person does not want a prayer, it is discourteous and alienating to impose one on them at their most vulnerable.

The guiding principle is to be 'person-centred'. Respect where the person is. It is no time to push your own views. Although many find comfort in a strong belief in a life after death, others with no such belief can prepare themselves for death equally well. Indeed, forms of belief, which involve a fear of agony in hell at the hands of the devil or a cruel God, can create an added dimension of terror. This kind of religion is increasingly under threat, even though some still approach their own death with a dread of severe punishment in the afterlife. Unforgiving fundamentalism still has an all too obvious, if bizarre, appeal in the world today.

RELIGION AND DEATH

Through religion, human beings have speculated widely about what, if anything, happens after death. Religious faith stretches the mind to its limits in the struggle to imagine the unimaginable: our possible survival outside the dimensions of time and space after our body (including our brain) has been destroyed. Some believe that human beings (and others that other animals also) survive individually in a kind of ethereal non-physical body. Others think that the soul survives in a disembodied form, while reincarnation in another body or identity makes sense to some. Yet another view is that we are absorbed into unity with all matter, losing any sense of our own individuality, while others remain convinced that death is without doubt the end of everything.

Many are clear only about their uncertainty: for them death is surrounded in mystery. As people involved in psychical research, medicine, physics, psychology and theology wrestle with the issue in different ways, the destiny for many is to die in doubt about life after death. For them, reflection leads to the refining of hope rather than belief.

On the other hand, many other people approach death confident that it is the gateway to something unimaginably positive and wonderful. C.S. Lewis described it at the end of his Narnia stories for children of all ages thus: 'All their life in this world and all their adventures in Narnia had only been the cover and the title page: now at last they were beginning Chapter One of the Great Story which no one on earth has read: which goes on forever: in which every chapter is better than the one before'.[7]

> Imelda, a shop manager, had retired from the company 10 years before but kept contact through a thriving company bridge club. After a series of strokes it became clear that she was dying. She had had a frustrating life in many ways, but she approached death with great serenity and optimism. Although she had not been much of a churchgoer and had no conventional belief in an afterlife, she felt that 'although I can't describe it, I know it's going to be alright'.

The sense that reality is ultimately benevolent, despite all the mixed messages of our existence, is the most hopeful response to the mystery of what may or may not come after death. On the other hand, others see the judgement of God, however merciful, after we die as necessary justice and ultimate accountability for what we do with our opportunities and talents. It has helped people endure the cruelty of tyrants. Faith or no faith, death can help us to reassess our values and priorities and sort out what is really important. Dr Johnson, the 18th century compiler of the first comprehensive English dictionary, wrote that being told that you will die in a fortnight 'wonderfully concentrates the mind'. John Brown, the American militant anti-slavery campaigner from Connecticut, was quoted as saying as he walked out to be executed in the American Civil War, that until that moment he had never fully realised how beautiful the world is.

SOME OF THE MAIN RELIGIOUS AND ATHEIST APPROACHES

In describing these, many sentences could be dotted with words that indicate not everyone who fits into this category believes exactly this or that! Within every 'ism' there is diversity. Every human being has a mind and heart with which to work out what they make of the world and their own experience, which is why they may start as one thing and end up as another. They may lose their faith or change their allegiance gradually or suddenly, like Paul on the road to Damascus. But there are plenty of disagreements within 'isms', some of which are both public and passionate, such as those about sexuality or whether war, terrorism or armed rebellion is justified. With that caveat, it may be helpful to have a little background on the 'ism' of the person you are trying to support if theirs is different to yours.

In a multicultural society, many people are exposed to the beliefs and practices around death in traditions other than their own. We also live in a world where more people are increasingly inclined to think things out for themselves rather than take the wisdom of the elders uncritically. Equally, the power of secularism and consumerism are also guiding many people, especially in the western world, away from traditional religious observance other than that of the replacement gods of shopping and entertainment.

While there are many similarities or overlap in beliefs and practice, people can and often do borrow ways of doing things from another belief system that makes sense to them. So, just as there are more mixed marriages, so there is more of a mixture of eclectic belief systems. This variety is illustrated in the following seven short sections, although in selecting them let me apologise to those readers who follow one of the many other faiths that I have failed to mention, as well as the limitations of what I have written about those that I have included.

Buddhism

In Buddhism, life is seen as a process of birth, ageing, illness and death, through which people may move towards enlightenment. We live and then we die. Whilst all physical manifestations of life must decline and disintegrate, life itself cannot be destroyed. Death is the time when a person's entity gathers energy to take on a new visible form. Physical appearance, followed by death, is the very rhythm of life itself. After death, life becomes a different form of energy, because energy is never destroyed. Energy is constant, even though physical matter changes every seven years. It is the energy that gives us a sense of continuity. Death changes the form of the energy from active to passive, not the energy itself. Death can thus be thought of as a period of latency, of passive life, just a different manifestation of life itself.

The body of a member of the family is traditionally kept at home for up to three days, when friends and relatives come to pay their respects with offerings of money or food. On the day of the funeral, the coffin is taken in procession, if possible, to the grave and a priest or monk is often asked to come to pray for the soul of the person who has died. On each anniversary of the death, to show respect to their memory, an offering of food is made on an altar in the home, dedicated to family ancestors.

Different schools of Buddhism have differences in practice. However Nichiren Daishonin (1222–1282) taught a daily practice through which people can draw forth their powerful inherent Buddha nature. In the Nichiren Buddhist school, for example, there are no priests or monks and funeral rites tend to take place in crematoria, conducted by a lay person. Two key chapters of the Lotus Sutra are recited, with the chanting of Nam myoho renge kyo, the same ceremony conducted daily each morning and evening. During the chanting, those who wish to can offer special powdered incense. As flowers are a symbol of impermanence, they are avoided. The altar is decorated with greenery and perhaps fruit, and guidance is given about the Buddhist view of death with readings from Nichiren Daishonin.[8]

Special chanting is conducted on the 7th, 49th and 100th day after death and thereafter on the subsequent anniversaries, particularly the 1st and 7th years, when an offering of food may be made on an altar in the home to show respect to their memory. This comes from a Japanese tradition called 'Urabon', recognising the various stages involved in death. The image is that of walking into the sea, shallow then deep, eventually stepping off the ledge to become fused with the universal life force of the universe. These ceremonies are an opportunity to show support to the bereaved and can be short and simple, though it has been known to have a glass of champagne to toast them.

Buddhism teaches that there are nine levels of consciousness: the ability to hear, see, smell, feel and taste are the first five; the 6th is our conscious mind, and the 7th – abstract thought and judgement – is active when we are both awake and asleep. The 8th level is where karma is stored during life, which becomes dominant over the other seven near to death. Karma is every function of our life: thoughts, words and deeds created through our other seven levels of consciousness. The 9th consciousness is the essence of universal and eternal life, which can potentially permeate the other eight levels. After our physical death, we remain in the state most strongly evoked in our karma, until our life becomes active again.[9]

Nirvana is an important concept in Buddhism, meaning literally extinction or quenching, and is the culmination of the spiritual journey for the truly enlightened person. Like the Christian idea of eternity, Nirvana is beyond, not after, death, because it is beyond or outside time and exists whether or not anyone attains it. Buddhists tend not to believe, however, in the survival of individual consciousness or awareness after death, the extinction of the 'fires' of attachment, hatred and delusion. Nirvana is the resultant state, which is beyond this world in the form of birth, ageing and death.[10]

Christianity

Christians traditionally believe in a life after death, although some are unsure. Heaven and hell were originally ideas from a pre-scientific concept of a three-tier universe, which made understanding much simpler: God was in heaven above the sky, hell was down below the flat earth and we lived out our lives in the middle. What has endured through our growing up scientifically is the belief that the destiny of human beings – at least – is to be with God in eternity, which is both outside time and space but may be experienced in flashes of transcendent experience in the present. As God is justice as well as compassion, we are judged for our behaviour and thoughts in relation to our love of God and neighbour, including our willingness to forgive others.

Justice requires us to take some responsibility for our behaviour and face up to its consequences somehow, even if we escape human justice. It requires a pattern of repentance and forgiveness, as a basis for own spiritual journey. That pattern, based on realistic rather than grovelling humility, is an essential ingredient of good relationships with other people, and for people with a faith, and with God. Judgement becomes fully apparent after or at the point of our death. For some, especially Catholics, after we die there is an intermediate stage called purgatory, in which we are purged of our sinfulness to the point where we are able to cope with being with God or not, as the case may be. Heaven would be hell if we cannot cope with the inescapable goodness and love of God, so they are not two places but different experiences of the same reality.

The ideas developed by Galileo Galilei (1564–1642) and other early scientists were beginning to influence how literally traditional beliefs could or should be understood. By the 18th century many European theologians came to doubt that there was literally such a place as hell (or heaven). Most of them did not rush to make this attitude public, however, since it was thought that the fear of damnation was essential to maintain public morality, a view many have sympathy with today![11] So eternity is now almost beyond human imagination tied as the latter to time and space. It is as mysterious and elusive as God is. Some Christians construct in their minds a parallel existence, in order to make sense of what happens when we die. Some science fiction plays with this concept, notably in the 1999 film *The Matrix*. As in many religions, there are, however, still many Christian fundamentalists who take the Bible to be literally true as far as they possibly can and regard much scientific thought as a threat rather than part of man's journey 'into all truth'.

The early Apostles Creed states succinctly that 'I believe in the resurrection of the body and the life everlasting'. Today, most orthodox Christian teaching continues to combine a belief in a life after death with that of liberation and 'new life' here and now, rather than 'pie in the sky when we die'. The conclusion remains, however, that 'it is not likely that there can emerge easily a Christian consensus on death and the after life, at any rate for a long time'.[12] Such a consensus is no more easily to be reached outside Christian circles.

For Christians, death is a time for grieving and celebration of the person's life, and this balance is often the aim of the funeral arrangements, which fit into the options described earlier in this chapter. Nevertheless, a danger for some Christians is to be so sure of the joy of being with God after death that grieving can be undermined and criticised as a lack of faith.

The various historical splits between the Christian churches, as with splits in other religions, have had a positive as well as a destructive element. They have enabled personal and cultural diversity to flower in a way that might have been more difficult in a unified church. Now that diversity is being belatedly honoured, the need for such splits as a means of the survival of religious integrity is becoming less pronounced. Hence the growth of the ecumenical movement, in which different churches and even different religions realise that what unites them is more important than what divides them and that their differences are more enriching and interesting than scandalous.

Hinduism

Gods in Hinduism are different manifestations of the Supreme Being, Brahman, whose existence is innate in everything that lives. Most Hindus believe in reincarnation, the nature of which is determined by the balance of good and bad deeds during their lifetime, so that life is a continuing flux of birth and rebirth. The souls of all living creatures are immortal. All life is sacred because God is in everything: to respect all life is to respect God. The combination of meditation, prayer and behaviour all combine to produce karma. Whatever evil is done comes back, if not in this life, in the way people are reborn. Karma continues through reincarnation.

The sacred Hindu scripture Bhagavad Gita (chapter 2: verses 18, 22 and 27) states: 'Finite they say are these our bodies indwelt by an eternal embodied soul – a soul indestructible. . . . As a man casts off his worn out clothes, and takes on other new ones in their place, so does the embodied soul cast off his worn out body and enters another anew. . . . For as sure is the death of all that comes to birth, sure the birth of all that dies'.

The Hindu who is ill or dying will want to hear readings from the sacred texts of the Bhagavad Gita, and may lie on the floor, close to Mother Earth. Traditionally, a priest will perform holy rites, perhaps blessing the person and sprinkling water on them (if possible from the River Ganges in India) to help the philosophical acceptance of death. Their relatives may also bring clothes and money for them to touch before being passed on to the needy.

Relatives are likely to accept death openly, which includes crying and expressing strong emotion. The body is conventionally prepared at home for the funeral, which, if possible, should take place within 24 hours of the death. Hindus tend to prefer cremation, although children and babies can be buried. The eldest male next-of-kin, who traditionally light the funeral pyre, collects the ashes on the 3rd day and takes them to scatter on water, ideally the river Ganges. Nowadays, modern forms of cremation are increasingly used.

Prayers are held in their home for the person who has died and immediate family and close friends attend these. These same people take it in
turns to provide a meal on each of the 31 days following death for all those
attending the prayers. At that point prayers at sunrise by the water, where
the ashes were scattered, signal the formal end of mourning. Further prayers
follow at home, followed by a celebratory meal. In Hinduism, prayers on
the anniversaries of the death are also important.

Humanism

'The mainsprings of moral action are what Darwin called the social instincts
– those altruistic, co-operative tendencies that are as much part of our
innate biological equipment as are our tendencies towards aggression and
cruelty.'[13] Humanists distance themselves from belief in God, religion or an
afterlife, with a focus on the human rather than a divine Spirit, and often
want to arrange for the funeral to be free from religious trappings. They are
often agnostic (not knowing if there is a God) or atheist (being sure that there
is no God). A humanist 'holds that man must face his problems with his
own intellectual and moral resources, without invoking supernatural aid'.[14]
Generally, humanists are sceptical about the value of religion, which is
essentially something that intelligent men and women are likely to outgrow,
especially if they can develop the maturity not to be dependent on its false
comforts. Some who grew up as religious may feel liberated and others a
poignant sense of loss, yet others a mixture of the two.

Much of the aesthetic heritage that religion has brought in terms of
music, art, architecture can, however, be enjoyed by and inspire many
humanists, whatever their culture. Some radical religious people, who take
all religious language to be symbolic rather than literal, can seem close
to humanists in what they believe. This can be a source of fruitful dialogue
or seen as an irritant in muddying what is thought should be clear water
between atheism and religion!

Non-specifically religious rituals are also now well established. The
British Humanist Association (see Appendix 4) can, for example, also
provide help with non-religious funerals. At a humanist funeral there is no
suggestion that the person has gone on to another life – it is the life that
was lived that is celebrated and the person people knew who is talked
about and said goodbye to. The Association has a network of accredited
officiants qualified to conduct humanist funerals.

Another ritual that has begun in the last decade or two in Britain is the
practice of creating a shrine in memory of a person who has died tragically.
Plaques in London have been put in the place where WPC Fletcher was
shot in 1984 while on duty during the Libyan Embassy siege and where
Stephen Lawrence was murdered in 1997 in an unprovoked racist attack.
Bunches of flowers are now frequently put in public places where people
have suddenly been killed, either through road accidents or murder, which
do not necessarily have any religious associations.

Islam

The Muslim faith was revealed to the prophet Mohammad. Although there are many cultural variations within Islam, Muslims have a strong belief in a life after death, which only separates us temporarily. There are different interpretations of the detail, some thinking that the body corrupts releasing the spirit and others that the body itself takes the spirit into the afterlife.

After death, the body should, if possible, be in the custody of Muslims. Normally only women wash a woman's body and men a man's. Any non-Muslim required to touch the body should wear disposable gloves. The body is dressed in a white shroud, called a Coffin, and should be buried, as was the prophet Mohammed, within 24 hours of dying, with the head facing in the direction of Mecca, the holy city of Islam. Grieving is often intense and uninhibited. Islam means surrender and most mourners in a Muslim ceremony, marked by urgency and spontaneity, believe in surrendering to the will of Allah as well as to how they feel. The funeral is simple with burial, if possible, in a Muslim cemetery and is still usually a man's affair, although women have started to accompany some funeral processions. It is a duty for family and friends to visit the bereaved.[15]

Many Muslims do not practice cremation, because of a belief that the body stays in the grave until God raises everyone from death on the Last Day to be judged, after which people will go for eternity to heaven or to hell.

Judaism

Judaism is reflected in different emphases, be it Orthodox, Progressive, Reform or Liberal. 'To everything there is a season: a time to be born, a time to die'. Judaism draws from biblical (what Christians call the Old Testament) and rabbinical texts, although how that material is interpreted for today, as with many religions, varies between conservative or orthodox and liberal or progressive movements. As with Christians and Muslims, some Jews believe in the resurrection of the dead, which is one of the 13 principles of faith set out by Maimonides. God will end the world when he decides to do so, creating a New World, a new Jerusalem and the Temple. Other Jews believe in a spirit world to which people go after death, rather than the idea of the Last Day.

Some Jews now choose cremation, although it used to be forbidden. Burial takes place as soon as possible and within three days of death. Coffins are simple and undecorated, so that no differentiation is made between rich and poor. If the cemetery is fairly accessible, the service begins in the chapel, which is stark, without flowers. A donation to a designated charity is the norm. Men and women usually stand apart at the service, in which there are psalms (especially Psalm 23), a memorial prayer and an eulogy in the local tongue.

Jewish cemeteries are called the House of Life, symbolising that death is not the end and that God will look after the faithful beyond the grave. The coffin is taken in procession, during which Psalm 91 is recited, to the grave.

The men attending fill the grave with soil. The shovel should not be passed from hand to hand, but replaced each time in the soil. The procession returns to the chapel, where everyone greets the mourners, before going back to the house of mourning, often that of the deceased, for a meal, prepared by others. There are customs to guide behaviour in the house of mourning, especially during the week of 'Shiva' following the funeral.

Visiting the sick is a religious duty (mitzvah) and it is important to pray and to work for the person's recovery, because of the sanctity of human life. 'Cast me not off in my old age when my strength fails, forsake me not. . . . But as for me, I will hope continually' (Psalm 71). Often a rabbi is wanted to help the dying person with prayer. A deathbed confession, where possible, helps to prepare for the next stage. The Mishnah puts it: 'The world is like an antechamber to the world to come; prepare thyself in the antechamber that thou mayest enter into the hall'.

After death, the treatment of the body is seen as a religious act and rules should be observed, preferably by trained volunteers of the same sex. Desecration of the body is forbidden in the Bible in the Book of Deuteronomy (chapter 21) and so post-mortems are not allowed unless the civil law requires it or if it is believed that an autopsy might save someone else.

As with people of other religious perspectives, the issue of mixed partnerships is impacting on Judaism: in the UK, for example, about half the Jewish people who are marrying are choosing a gentile. Traditionally, only Jews could be buried in a Jewish cemetery, although consideration is now being given in some liberal circles to the possibility of a couple from a mixed marriage being buried together in a Jewish cemetery.

There is little about life after death in the Jewish Bible, which emphasises this life. However, rabbinical teaching developed a concept of the immortality of the soul and even the resurrection of the dead. So Judaism has been described as both this- and other-worldly. This paradox is illustrated when the 2nd century Rabbi Jacob wrote: 'Better is one hour of repentance and good deeds in this world than the whole life of the world to come; yet better is one hour of blissfulness of spirit in the world to come than the whole life of this world'.[16]

Sikhism

Sikhism, like Hinduism, advances belief in reincarnation. A person's life cycle depends on how their present life is lived, although everyone is born in the grace of God. Life is mortal but the spirit is immortal. Some Sikhs are confirmed by taking 'Amrit', after which they should attend the temple daily for prayer and wear five symbols, the 'Ks': Keshas – uncut hair, Kangha – the comb, Kara – a steel bangle, Kirpan – a short sword, and Kaachh – a pair of shorts as underwear. These symbols, especially the hair, wherever possible, should not be removed in life or after death.

Reciting hymns from the Guru Granth Sahib will comfort a dying Sikh. If they are not well enough, a relative, a reader from the local temple or even another practising Sikh does this. Relatives prefer as far as possible to be with the person as they die. Although it is also usually acceptable for non-Sikhs to tend to the body, the family should be asked if they wish to wash and lay it out. The body is normally displayed at home prior to cremation for friends and relatives to view. Sikhs are always cremated, if possible within 24 hours, and the ashes if possible scattered in a river, preferably the Ganges. Funeral rites, with a procession to the crematorium, are important. When attending funerals, women usually wear a white head covering. For about 10 days after the funeral, relatives gather for the completion of the reading of the holy book, the Guru Granth Sahib, either at home or the Gurdwara or temple.

WORKING WITH YOUR OWN EXPERIENCES

What seems to help many people come to terms with death is for them to have faith or, as it originally means, trust in the situation in which they find themselves. This may involve them trying to work out, in the light of experience, what they believe about death and come up with their own conclusions, however tentative. They may, however, put their trust in an existing religious or non-religious position, because they trust the people who espouse it and accept its teaching. Whether or not this takes them to a religious or an agnostic position, orthodox or unorthodox, may be secondary. The people who sometimes find it harder to cope with death are those who have avoided the issue, as if it was too terrifying or depressing to contemplate. Their sense of being at sea in the face of death may be acute, and their need for support may consequently be greater and the support that they receive all the more crucial.

Notes

1 Brady, D. (2003) 'Mourning in America: an interview with Katherine Ashenburg', *BusinessWeek*, 23 October. See also: Ashenburg, K. (2003) *The Mourner's Dance*, New York, NY: North Point Press.
2 Knight, M. (1961) *Humanist Anthology from Confucius to Bertrand Russell*, London: Barrie & Rockliff for The Rationalist Press.
3 Murray Parkes, C., Laungani, P. and Young, B. (eds) (1996) *Death and Bereavement across Cultures*, London: Routledge.
4 Moss, B. (2002) 'Spirituality: a personal view', in N. Thompson (ed) (2002) *Loss and Grief: A Guide for Human Services Practitioners*, Basingstoke: Palgrave.
5 Lloyd, M. (1997) 'Dying and bereavement, spirituality and social work in a market economy of welfare', *British Journal of Social Work*, vol 27, no 2: 175–90.
6 Lewis, C.S. (1960) *The Four Loves*, London: Geoffrey Bless.
7 Lewis, C.S. (1956) *The Last Battle*, London: The Bodley Head.
8 Baynes, A. (1992) *What Happens When We Die?*, Taplow Court, Berkshire.
9 Daisaku, I. (2003) *Unlocking the Mysteries of Birth and Death*, 2nd ed. Santa Monica, California: Middleway Press.
10 His Holiness the Dalai Lama (1996) *The Good Heart*, London: Rider.

11 Smart, N. (1968) 'Death in the Judaeo-Christian tradition', in A. Toynbee
     Man's Concern with Death, London: Hodder & Stoughton.
12 Smart, N. (1968), *ibid.*
13 Knight, M. (1961), *ibid.*
14 Knight, M. (1961), *ibid.*
15 Collins, D., Tank, M. and Basith, A. (1992) *Concise Guide to Customs of Minority
     Ethnic Religions*, Portsmouth: Portsmouth Diocesan Council for Social
     Responsibility.
16 Jacobs, L. (1973) *What does Judaism Say About?*, Jerusalem: Keter.

The workplace, death and bereavement

Chapter 12

Is it any of our business?

- 'Least said, soonest mended'
- Emotional literacy and leadership
- Loss, change and transition
- Barriers breaking down between work and personal life
- Support and motivation

'LEAST SAID, SOONEST MENDED?'

Most managers and other people at work do not expect to deal with bereavement or terminal illness as part of the 'day job'. It may not crop up for years, but when it does, it can hit home all too suddenly. The manager can feel that it is hardly part of the job description, training or experience and can consequently feel out of their depth. Alternatively and even worse, they may have no idea of the degree to which they are putting their foot in it. For the person or people affected, this is likely to be a crucial time in their lives at which they plumb depths of possibly unfamiliar, profound and probably painful feelings and experiences. Helping to provide good support is the intention of this book, so that we are no longer at a loss over grief in the workplace; but the rationale for this cannot be taken for granted.

Death and dying can all too easily be thought of as largely part of the post-retirement agenda, and that it should not intrude embarrassingly into the great priorities of taking the business forward. Even in a hospital setting, a core member of the team ringing in because someone close to them has died can feel like an irritation. The streak in our culture that wishes to ignore or at least sideline death runs deep. At least 500 years ago a proverb was coined: 'Neither for peace nor for warre, will a dead bee gather honey'. In the hive, a bee's remains are meticulously removed, so that there is no 'dead space', and then they are discarded. Likewise, in terms of output, the dead employee is unproductive. If the deceased is the partner, parent or child of one of our colleagues, they can be of no further use to the company as a staff supporter or motivator. 'Let the dead bury their dead', Jesus is reported to have said. That life is for living and for the living is a principle followed in the natural world, where many animals quickly ignore the corpse of a member of their own family, unless it is regarded as edible. There are exceptions, especially among some mammals: elephants, for example, sometimes stay with the body or bones of a member of their group and engage in behaviour that looks to human eyes very like grieving.

If we concentrate on the bottom line, it might seem that we should cut our losses, or at least minimise any further investment, human or financial, for the dying and bereaved. Pension and insurance arrangements and an adequate compassionate leave policy should cover it; with a note of sympathy, a floral tribute or contribution to a chosen charity and perhaps attendance at the funeral.

The resource implications of doing more may be greater than we first imagine: according to CRUSE, the bereavement care agency, about 3,500 people are newly bereaved in the UK each day and one person loses their partner every three minutes. A work–life balance survey carried out by the British Department of Trade and Industry identified that 'equally 14% of male and 14% of female employees had taken bereavement leave in the 12 month period'.[1]

Grieving is not necessarily open to a quick fix. The bereaved often need ongoing thoughtful support over a period of weeks or months, rather than days. For some people, the feelings associated with death are embarrassing, and can cause us to feel uncomfortable. Bereavement can undermine years of conditioning in the British stiff upper lip. Hence the perceived need for tight control. No wonder Geoffrey Gorer, in his study *Death, Grief and Mourning*,[2] concluded that 'giving way to grief is stigmatised as morbid, unhealthy, demoralising. The proper action of a friend and well wisher is felt to be the distraction of a mourner from his or her grief'. Forty years after that was written, such an attitude is still widespread, even though a more enlightened and open attitude is becoming more common. In America, it has been suggested, for example, that 'in practice even employee-focused organisations find dealing with employees who have suffered a loss among the most awkward, and least talked about work-related topics'.[3]

Whereas sex was the great taboo for the Victorians, for much of the 20th century it was replaced by death. Sex has often been promoted to symbolise health, happiness, eternal youth and success in our culture. Death, on the other hand, can be seen as representing the opposite of life, as well as being one of the realities that is most dreaded, despite or perhaps because of its inevitability. No wonder that it is seen as negative, depressing or demoralising, for many best avoided and can so easily become an 'undiscussable'.

There are, however, occasions when no one can dodge bereavement at work. September 11th 2001 in America was, for example, one of these. The World Trade Center was targeted by terrorists because it was a workplace, albeit one of a particular significance. The planes that were hijacked and flown into it were originally piloted and staffed by people at work. Many of the passengers were travelling on business. The fire fighters, police and others who died in the rescue attempts were at work. They demonstrated so courageously what the commitment of people in those lines of work can cost. The attacks were designed to create as many traumatic bereavements as possible, as well as heightening the anticipatory fear of being killed going to or being at work. What terrorism continues to bring to work is the sense that virtually anyone may be killed in the course of duty, a sense that in the past was restricted to jobs that were clearly dangerous. To keep matters in perspective, however, it has been pointed out that whereas three thousand died on September 11th, at least that number died on the beaches of Normandy. 'Sixty million died in all between 1939 and 1945. The annual average number of casualties from terrorism world-wide over the past five years, even including September 11th, is around a thousand.'[4]

EMOTIONAL LITERACY AND LEADERSHIP

Attitudes are, however, changing. This is part of a broader recognition of the importance of emotional intelligence at work replacing the idea that feelings and intelligence are opposites and almost mutually exclusive.[5] That approach saw feelings as largely out of place at work, because they stopped people thinking clearly and logically. So a culture was encouraged in which the acknowledgement and expression of feelings, especially among men, was restricted as far as possible to home. It started at school and continued at work, from the armed services to factories and offices through to hospitals. The old stereotype that men are unemotional and intelligent and women are the opposite is under concerted attack in the face of evidence as opposed to prejudice. Sport was something of a halfway house in which boys and men were allowed an outlet for their passion and exuberance: that trend gathers apace. The handshakes and smiles of yesterday are replaced today by the hugs and whoops of triumph when the goal is scored, the wicket taken. Enlightened coaches, who know that enthusiasm endorse this and commitment can be increased through their expression. Of course there are still many, in sport, parenting and teaching as well as in the workplace, who sing to a different tune: all stick and minimum carrot. 'Don't waste time and breathe, conserve it for the essential task of showing them where they have got it wrong.' Good managers, as part of their responsibility for motivation, also realise how important it is to encourage and praise their staff not only for achievements but also for effort.

There seem to be five interrelated strands of thought behind these changing attitudes:

- Feelings are closely related to the energy, enthusiasm and motivation needed at work.
- Within feelings and intuition, there may be important information that a business is unwise to ignore.
- Emotional intelligence is often an essential ingredient to building good working relationships.

- Feelings are part of our humanity and deserve to be valued, as well as managed, rather than belittled.
- Human character traits traditionally associated with women are less likely to be discounted now as a result of changing attitudes in society towards women, among both men and women.

People at work who are comfortable with their feelings and those of other people are more likely to respect and be interested in the feelings that are associated with bereavement and affect behaviour and performance.

A key underpinning for any effective support in any of these roles is empathy, which, along with respect and genuineness, is considered further in Appendix 2. It can be thought of as the balancing between sympathy and apathy, avoiding the dangers of both, although sympathy has of course an honourable place in supporting those who are bereaved, but it has its dangers.

The empathy continuum

Sympathy   - the danger of over-involvement and being so sorry for the person that they may feel patronised and more depressed.

Empathy   - communicating understanding of the way that they experience the world, death and bereavement; the balance between sympathy and apathy.

Apathy   - lack of involvement, indifference, uncaring, emotionally distant.

Empathy used to be widely regarded as of little concern outside counselling and psychotherapy. It is now increasingly being realised as fundamental to any good relationship, at home or work. A leading consultant, Dr. Peter Drucker, has identified it as a critical aspect of management, and Dr. David Freemantle is among those who have recently argued that 'senior executives, middle managers and supervisors need to demonstrate "genuine heart-felt" empathy for their various teams of employees. When you have a senior boss who feels *warm* about his or her people and whom they, in turn, feel warm about, then an organisation will develop a *warm* culture (as opposed to a *cold* one). All the progressive organisations I have studied around the world in the research for my various books are now moving towards a *warm* culture based on empathy. They are going beyond efficiency to *add emotional value (AEV)* in all their dealings with employees, customers and suppliers alike'.[6]

LOSS, CHANGE AND TRANSITION

For a business to prosper, it is crucial that change is managed effectively. To do that, people are needed who can cope with transition at all levels, including the personal. Bereavement is one example of loss and although it is the focus of this book, it will not be difficult for the reader to relate what is written to other experiences of loss. An occupational health nurse of a chemical company, for example, told me that in her work the two big personal issues that members of staff were bringing to her that were really sabotaging their ability to focus on their work were bereavement and divorce. The latter was a major loss, involving the need to come to terms and to grips with the death of a relationship.

Most change involves both loss and gain, while the ultimate losses are those of our own life or of those closest to us. Consequently, the ability to cope with the death of others may well help us to manage other lesser losses, including those at work. Conversely, unresolved loss in one area of our life may make subsequent changes difficult to manage, even where the link between the two may not be obvious.

Colin Maxwell[7] wrote that 'The Jungian view of growth through loss has great relevance in terms of bereavement in the workplace. It offers an ideal opportunity for organisations to demonstrate their caring style of management. If they fail on this issue, the disillusion and bitterness that they reap can be great and long lasting. On the other hand, bereavement can cut through social and organisational barriers, through custom and practice. It reminds us of our common humanity and makes differences between us seem irrelevant and superficial'. A caring style of management may sound sentimental to some, but it should not. It is rather a passionate commitment to the task and to the people. If the company does not care about me at such a time, why should I care about the success of the company?

> Peter, a 43-year-old sales manager, was made redundant in October. He was a resilient person who had responded positively and enthusiastically to change in the company over the years, seeing it as a challenge. His senior management predicted that he would cope well with the redundancy: he was one of many and therefore need not take it personally, and his prospects for re-employment were excellent because of his good reputation and contacts. But his employers had not taken into account the implications of a double bereavement: his mother had died four months before and his wife a year previously. At the time, he had apparently taken their deaths 'amazingly well, considering' and had carried on 'almost as if nothing had happened'. The culture in the company did little to encourage the grieving process and redundancy was the last straw. It felt to him as if his world, already crumbling, had finally crashed. Before he could give his attention to the job search, he had to attend to his grief and begin to reconstruct a world in which going for a job made some kind of sense.

In Peter's case, he had some bereavement counselling, which concentrated on the deaths of the two most important women in his life. After a few sessions he was able to refocus on the job search successfully and function effectively at interviews. His psychological resources had virtually run dry by the time the redundancy occurred. If he had been made redundant before the bereavements, he would have probably taken it in his stride.

As children we sometimes have two perceptions of the world: one, a sense that we will never die; the other, a feeling that the world about us does not or should not change. Both attitudes usually change with age, but their echoes can linger in nostalgia. As a consequence, we can feel resentful if our organisation does not keep things as they are or used to be, even though adult realism indicates that the world is in a constant state of flux, as we are, and companies that do not adapt, perish.

We need to recognise and come to terms with this tension, learning to accept and even, where appropriate, to welcome change. This is preferable to trying to block it, like someone who tries to fight the ageing process instead of growing old gracefully. The death of someone close to us is about the most challenging change some people are ever likely to face.

BARRIERS BREAKING DOWN BETWEEN WORK AND PERSONAL LIFE

Erecting mental barriers between our personal and work lives is a common way of managing both. At work, we may get respite from family pressures and vice versa. We need to let our concerns in one area go, so that we can concentrate on the other. These intrinsically useful barriers may, however, be negatively reinforced if people at work are treated as if their life outside work neither exists nor matters. A way of coping with this is to try and split life into two: at work being whole-hearted about the job, but at home being all for the family and 'never the twain shall meet'.

But the whole person is there in both aspects of our life, notably in our capacity to learn, develop and mature. The impact of a significant death is so great that it cannot be ignored either at work or home: a rigid split becomes particularly difficult to sustain in this instance. Even if the bereaved person may want to use work to try and forget a little, it is often impossible to draw a line around it.

A good employer does not reinforce the split between life at work and life outside work, because they will intrude into each other. Successes and significant events, such as births as well as deaths, need to be recognised and, where appropriate, allowed for.

SUPPORT AND MOTIVATION

Those who are helped to work through bereavement are more likely to be able to give support to colleagues who face major difficulties. On the other hand, if bereavement has not been adequately dealt with, there may be continuing problems in an individual's relationship to work. These can include, for example, lack of concentration, reduced interest and motivation, depression, displaced anger and irritability.

A common response to a bereavement is that it is a time 'when you find out who your real friends are'. These are the people who not only care but who also, through their skills and sensitivity, avoid 'putting their foot in it'. A bereaved person, exceptionally vulnerable and in a state of heightened awareness, can be simultaneously both appreciative and also critical of other people's responses. He or she may view other people in the extreme as either good or bad, and the same can apply to a company. If others are experienced as a source of help rather than hindrance, long-term goodwill has been won and the ripples from that will have a positive impact on other employees who observe, maybe discreetly, how a colleague was treated at such a time.

> The young wife of Colin, a market researcher in a packaging company, died after a protracted battle against a malignant disease. The personal support of his departmental head was crucial to his recovery. He gave Colin time to talk through how things were going and reassured him that he need not worry about work at such a time. The concern continued to be expressed for months, thus making him feel that he was not under pressure to behave 'as if nothing had happened'. The support which that manager (and through him the company) had given at such a traumatic time in his life strengthened Colin's loyalty and commitment to them both.

Goodwill can thus reach beyond the person immediately affected. This is true whether the employee is dying or is bereaved. Others will draw their own conclusions about the quality of support (or lack of it) that they and their families might receive in such a crisis themselves. An organisation's support needs to flow from a serious commitment to staff, rather than seeing people merely as instruments for exploitation and securing profits. These messages flow out of the company to customers and even suppliers. A concern for ethical investment includes how staff are treated, wherever the company operates. It is no use having framed *Investors in People* certificates in reception, if the organisation is experienced as callous and insensitive when staff or clients are at their most vulnerable.

If we want the whole-hearted support of staff to their work and to the company, that commitment has to be reciprocal. We need to be committed to them as human beings, not as units of production or disembodied brains or 'hands' to be exploited without feeling. Bereavement is often an over-whelming experience and can and does happen to any of us. A manager committed to a staff member cannot ignore their needs at such a time, and should be concerned to provide appropriate support.

The case for the company to provide committed and informed support can therefore be justified on a variety of grounds. The Work Foundation suggested that 'employers and organisations who manage the situation effectively when employees are dealing with death and bereavement befit in a number of ways as the employees who feel supported by an understanding manager will maintain better working relationships, and are less likely to lose motivation or productivity'.[8]

Notes

1 Department of Trade and Industry (2000) *Work–life Balance Survey*, appendix F, London: DTI.
2 Gorer, G. (1965) *Death, Grief and Mourning*, London: Crescent.
3 Robinson-Jacobs, K. (2000) 'No longer at loss over grief in the workplace', *Los Angeles Times*, 13 June.
4 The Observer (1904) *Why we remember (D-Day)*, London: The Observer, 6 June.
5 Bagshaw, M. (2000) *Using Emotional Intelligence at Work*, Ely: Fenman.
6 Freemantle, D. (1998) *What Customers Like about You*, London: Nicholas Brealey Publishing.
7 Maxwell, C. 'Bereavement counselling', *Journal of Workplace Learning*, vol 5, no 2.
8 The Work Foundation (2002) *Training Pack – Bereavement Issues in the Workplace*, London: The Work Foundation.

Chapter 13

How the organisation can help

- Organisational culture, atmosphere and core values
- Compassionate leave policy
- Payments of benefits following death
- Carers
- Induction and training
- An in-service staff support network
- Bereavement counselling

The employer has a significant role in the bereavement process:

- in representing part of wider society;
- in providing a place to mourn or sometimes a place to escape from grieving;
- in being a bridge between grief and returning to 'normality'.

ORGANISATIONAL CULTURE, ATMOSPHERE AND CORE VALUES

The experience of bereavement or terminal illness concentrates the mind on what is really important. The need to feel that work is of value to society as well as a means of making money often comes to the fore in answer to the question: why bother? Of course, even the most inspiring work can be reduced to drudgery by the touch of death. The sense that the organisation cares about its people, customers and staff, and not only about money, however that may be measured, is important at such a time.

For some, caring is a tricky word, carrying in its trail charges of hypocrisy, sentimentality or being unbusiness-like. But whatever euphemism is used, the concept is fundamental to a company's responsibility for the individual. Any organisation needs a culture in which staff are valued for their humanity, not just as units of production to be mercilessly exploited. How a bereavement is handled will reflect that culture, hopefully for good rather than ill.

With the need for companies to avoid being bureaucratic and rigid, corporate values and style tend to replace explicit rules and policies as a more flexible way of holding the company together and giving it an identity. If the values are thought to be just bits of paper that do not reflect how people really try to behave, especially those at the top, the result, however, is cynicism and a belief that the company is hypocritical, in which case they are counterproductive.

On the other hand, a strong sense of a shared direction can help raise morale and promote motivation: 'A vision without a task is a dream: a task without a vision is drudgery'. Good values need to be promoted with determination, and checked out with good listening and other mechanisms, such as staff attitude surveys or 360 degree feedback. An enlightened organisation is one in which people feel that they can be themselves, take risks and be messengers of bad as well as good news without fear. Those characteristics of not having to pretend can help the business face up to and address problems, rather than ignoring them until it is too late. They can also help create a climate in which it feels relatively safe to be vulnerable personally as well as professionally.

The Work Foundation, formerly The Industrial Society,[1] has put the relationship between the different terms as follows:

- A *Vision* is our ultimate aim.
- The *Mission* is the purpose for which we exist.
- Our core *Values* are the beliefs which we hold that guide our day-to-day behaviour, actions and decisions.

The atmosphere of a workplace has been described as a very subtle group presence. John O'Donoghue wrote that 'It is difficult to describe or analyse an ethos; yet you immediately sense its power and effect. Where it is positive, wonderful things can happen. It is a joy to come to work, because the atmosphere comes out to meet you, and it is a happy atmosphere. It is caring, kind and creative. Where the ethos of the workplace is negative and destructive, people wake up in the morning and the first thought of going to work literally makes them ill'.[2] Many workplaces fall somewhere in between, depending on events and personalities as well as the attitudes that trickle down from directors and managers at every level.

A positive atmosphere does not preclude conflict or anger, but it does enable disagreements to be managed constructively. Conflict can be managed more or less constructively and anger channelled so that abuse and bullying are minimised, if not avoided. Enlightened leaders, from chief executives to first-line managers, team leaders and supervisors, appreciate that it is part of their job to help create such an atmosphere in the interests of productivity and innovation as well as morale.[3] To do so requires skill as well as commitment, but is an important ingredient in developing people who are motivated and focused.

With respect to death and bereavement, a supportive, enabling organisational culture is obviously more appropriate in helping staff cope with bereavement than a blaming, punitive one. The most relevant and vital values guiding day-to-day behaviour are those of:

- genuineness
- understanding through active noticing and listening
- mutual respect for people irrespective of their status or seniority.

(These are discussed more fully in Appendix 2: 'The core conditions of helping'.)

The starting point can be one of encouragement. In a recent study, many people who have been bereaved found that work was helpful during their bereavement, even though a lesser number did not, finding it an added dimension of distress and stress.[4] In 1998, however, Sue Shellenberger wrote in the Wall Street Journal that 'bereavement is a blind spot for many bosses and workers. Though understanding of the grieving process has advanced light years in recent decades, workplace attitudes are stuck in the Industrial Age'.[5] Elsewhere it is argued that death was less of a taboo in the west in the 19th than the 20th centuries.

A modern organisational approach that is helpful in supporting people at work to cope with bereavement or terminal illness will include:

- an unequivocal commitment to staff as a resource rather than a cost even though following a bereavement they are may be less productive than usual;
- a commitment to support employees during bereavement, recognising that bereaved staff who are well supported by their employer and subsequently work through their grief well, will invariably grow in the process and strengthen their loyalty to the company;
- a commitment to people in the whole of their lives, recognising that the quality of life outside work is relevant to their contribution at work.

And a company culture in which:

- open and honest communication is encouraged;
- the difference between direct feedback and attacking colleagues is understood;
- bullying, abuse and inappropriate fear is unacceptable;[6]
- human vulnerability is respected, and not despised as a weakness;
- feelings and their expression, including tears, are seen as part of our humanity rather than just as a cause of embarrassment;
- a management style is promoted, which takes account of the human needs of and pressures on staff (and their families) and has respect for a healthy 'work-life' balance between time and commitment to work and life outside work.

COMPASSIONATE LEAVE POLICY

The need for flexibility around compassionate leave has been widely argued and almost as widely accepted. Another article by Sue Shellenbarger, for example, argued that 'a death in today's far-flung families can mean a 3,000 mile trip just to get to the funeral, requiring extended time off. And as the definition of *family* changes, the loss of a housemate or friend can be just as devastating to an employee's productivity and morale as the death of a parent'.[7] A survey, published in Britain two years later by The Work Foundation, found that nearly all (99%) of the respondents stated that employees are allowed time off for bereavement, although it is only automatically paid for in 58% of the sample of 503 organisations. In a piece of unwelcome discrimination, a tiny 1% only paid for white collar workers. Almost as disappointing are the 2% who refuse pay for all employees. The leave tends to be a mixture of paid and unpaid for 37% of organisations, which is sensible if the approach is sufficiently flexible.[8] However, another study suggested that more employees are unaware of their organisation's bereavement policies than those who are aware of them.[9]

How flexible is it possible to be, given the needs of both the company and member of staff? The message a bereaved staff member needs to hear initially is that work comes second even though it is important: they must take what time out is needed. Situations vary depending on circumstances and personalities: some want to come back relatively soon after the funeral, while others need more time off. What is not helpful, for example as in one case, is a note on their return curtly telling them that they have exceeded their leave entitlement and should get an annual leave application in urgently.

Compassionate leave policy needs to be flexible and generous, with the line manager having a delegated discretion to offer more than the minimum if it seems warranted. Such leave should be available over a period and not restricted to the time before and immediately after the funeral. This can be usefully codified in the organisation formulating and negotiating a flexible return to work policy that can be applied in some bereavements as well as in some cases of illness. It may also be relevant during a person's terminal illness and not only after they have died. In the UK, section 57A of the Employment Rights Act 1996 gave an employee a statutory right to take a reasonable amount of unpaid time off in a variety of circumstances:

a)   to provide assistance when a dependant falls ill, gives birth, is injured or assaulted;

b)   to make arrangements for the care of a dependant who is ill or injured;

c)   in consequence of the death of a dependant;

d)   because of the unexpected disruption or termination of arrangements for the care of a dependant;

e)   to deal with an incident that involves a child of the employee and which occurs unexpectedly when the child is at school.

The right to apply requires the employee to tell the employer the reason for their absence as soon as is practicable and how long he or she expects to be absent, unless he has already returned. The Work Foundation has elaborated on this helpfully in its management factsheet on compassionate leave.[10]

Leave arrangements rightly judged benefit the company as well as the individual. Someone at work who is emotionally absent and distracted, let alone distraught, may with a little more judiciously judged phased leave become someone who can contribute really effectively again. Dr. Kenneth Doka, the professor of gerontology at the College of New Rochelle in New York, has been quoted as saying: 'One of the things we do know about grief is it does affect your judgement, and you do not process information as quickly, and are more likely to make cognitive mis-steps'.[11] While executives may have good coping skills, they need to be aware of their limitations in such circumstances.

> In a Young Offenders Unit, the inmates could only have compassionate leave to attend the funeral in the case of parents or siblings, not for grandparents, who in some cases happened to be the adults to whom they were closest. An imaginative chaplain offered a parallel service in the chapel at the same time as the funeral.

A family can be defined as those you care for and who care for you and compassionate leave is increasingly encompassed under the broader heading of Family Leave. This will include parental, maternal and paternal, and adoption leave as well as a more general heading of leave for family reasons. Under the latter heading, the Trades Union Congress (TUC) includes death and such other pressing reasons as the illness of a spouse, elderly relative, child or person looking after a child, a child's wedding, as well as caring for partners, dependants and individuals in stable relationships though not related by marriage or blood.[12]

Organisations vary, as the examples below illustrate, as to how prescriptive they are. In the first example, a close relative could be interpreted narrowly or more flexibly to include an unmarried partner, gay or heterosexual, or even a very close friend. Companies attempting a detailed list need to include unmarried partners if they are serious about their commitment to equality of opportunity.

None of the examples mentions specifically the death of colleagues, even though a number of staff would be expected to attend the funeral in such an event, and it would normally take place during working hours.

A large national utility also provided its staff with a list as a guideline, which included grandchildren, brother-in-law, sister-in-law, son-in-law and daughter-in-law. In this organisation, for some of these categories, paid leave for a funeral was only to be granted if the relative shared the same house as the staff member. Lists can be helpful as guidelines, but also woefully inadequate to deal with the complex reality of human relationships if they are always applied rigidly.

Examples of company policy in relation to bereavement:

Example 1. Time off: introductory comments

If urgent private matters require your attention at any time you should apply for leave of absence to your senior. Such requests are always considered sympathetically. Management will generally be fairly tolerant to requests for occasional days off (normally without pay) for family reasons and a more disciplined approach towards other personal business which can normally be arranged on pre-arranged 'days off'. It is essential that you give as much notice as possible.

There are people with no close relatives or, if they do exist, are so alienated that they do not even come to the funeral, let alone organise it. In such circumstances, this and related responsibilities may fall to a friend, who might in turn also happen to be a colleague. Friends can be closer than family, which is why the word 'normally' needs to be in the 2nd sentence of the next example to accommodate some flexibility.

Example 2. Bereavement

Where an employee is personally responsible for the funeral arrangements of a close relative, up to 3 days' leave may be granted with pay. This will only apply at the time of the bereavement, however, and is restricted to close relatives.

Example 3. Bereavement leave

An employee is eligible for up to 3 days' leave with pay in respect of the death of an immediate relative or dependant, who is defined as spouse, son, daughter, parent, brother, sister and also includes common-law spouse and legally adopted children. In the event of the death of a grandparent, grandchild or in-law, the employee may be granted paid leave to attend the funeral.

Example 4. Leave of absence to attend funerals of near relatives

Leave with pay will, normally not exceeding one day, be granted to members of staff to enable them to attend the funeral of a wife or husband, child, father, mother, step-father, step-mother, brother, sister, step-brother, step-sister, mother-in-law, father-in-law, grandfather, grandmother, and the spouses of a grandfather/a grand-mother. In the case of other near-relatives, staff will be allowed to change their turn of duty, where practicable, to enable them to attend the funeral.

The company has indicated that when an employee is the sole member of the family responsible for making all the arrangements in connection with the funeral, the local manager can, at his or her discretion, grant leave with pay up to a total of five days, if considered necessary.

Time off to attend funerals (see also Chapter 10) in work time is sometimes given to attend any funeral, particularly for those of former colleagues, without requiring the member of staff to take annual leave. However, this is seldom laid down as company policy but rather seen as discretionary.

While there are stories of the person who goes to an impossible number of grandmothers' funerals, a caring manager who asks sensitively after the person will come to realise how emotionally close the person is to the one who has died. It is the level of emotional closeness, rather than the formal relationship, that generally determines the level of mourning the staff member will experience. The impact of the tragic death in 2002 of the England cricketer Ben Hollioake illustrates this. Alec Stewart wrote: 'It was an awful moment. I hadn't just lost a valued teammate, but far more importantly a close friend and a great bloke. The Surrey players all flew out to Perth [in Australia] for the service and funeral. It was a sombre flight'.[13]

Figures from the UK Labour Research Department's 1997 database report reveal that, on average, an employee will receive five days' paid leave after the death of a member of their immediate family (partner, parent, child or sibling) and two days for other family members. In many companies this is the extent of the support,[14] reinforcing the notion that bereavement is a five-day event or even less, as of course it may be where the friendship or emotional connection has been minimal. Many relationships, however, at work as well as outside work go much deeper. Such depth contributes to the effectiveness of many individuals and teams, who excel through their commitment and passion. Sting expressed the depth of the impact of some deaths when he spoke of John Lennon on the 20th anniversary of his death: 'What happens when people like that die is that the landscape changes. You know, a mountain disappears, a river is gone. And I think that his death was probably as significant as that'.[15] The landscape changes for many people after the deaths of many less famous. The empathic manager will sense that when it happens in others, if not necessarily in him- or herself.

PAYMENTS OF BENEFITS FOLLOWING DEATH

The prompt payments of benefits, including shares, can be difficult if no specification has been made. Companies need to try to ensure that such payments go to the right person, especially dependants, such as partner and children, including adopted ones, who are under the age of 18 or still receiving full-time education or training. Where there is a dispute or lack of clarity about who is entitled, the employer needs to consult the person's legal representative.

CARERS

A bigger challenge for organisations arises in the case of long-term sickness of someone in a close relationship in which a staff member becomes the main carer. An estimated 20% of the six million people in the UK who care for frail elderly, seriously ill or disabled people at home are also in full-time employment and many others work away from the home part time. By 2011, the estimate for the number of carers will have increased to 13 million, with a corresponding greater impact on people at work directly and indirectly.[16] Not surprisingly many carers get depressed from time to time, as it is often depressing work: 80% of them are thought to have suffered depression and as many as a third have not had a break for over two years. When people become terminally ill, this need may continue for a matter of weeks or months, and a great deal of flexibility may be asked of the employer, from regular or irregular shorter or flexible hours to significant periods of extended leave, paid or unpaid.

The TUC and the Carers National Association have produced a useful *Charter for Carers*:[17]

- Caring is difficult, demanding, and requires high levels of professional skills.
- Carers' own needs are important.
- Trades unions should oppose employment discrimination against carers and part-time workers.
- The TUC calls for adequately funded 'care in the community' without delay.
- The TUC calls for government funding for support services for frail, elderly and disabled people, especially respite care. There should be sufficient provision to give all frail and disabled people a right to the support of professional carers.
- Trades unions should seek to negotiate flexible working packages from employers, including the same pay and benefits, pro rata, as for other employees.
- Unions should press for a right for carers who have to give up work to return without loss of any employment rights.
- Training and retraining for carers and former carers returning to the labour market should be another union priority.
- Invalid Care Allowance should be extended to everyone who cares for another adult for 35 hours a week or more.
- The TUC calls for a statutory right to special leave.

An employer can help staff decide how to attend to the urgent and often distressing responsibility of ensuring that their nearest and dearest are adequately cared for when they can no longer look after themselves. While admission into a care or nursing home may be the 'least worst' solution, it may be that care at home is the preferred option. In that event, it may include the carer going part time, working flexibly or giving up their former job for a period. In that event, if the option of coming back to work later is kept open, it is likely to provide a considerable measure of comfort and perhaps affirmation, if they are really valued. They will also need their line manager's sensitive support even if they are able to continue to work and their working hours do not change.

The way the work is organised does not always make flexibility an option for the carer, but it is always worth looking at what might be possible. Martin, for example, talks about the support he received from his boss, after his wife had been diagnosed with advanced cancer:

> I used to think that my boss didn't manage people very well; but when the chips were down and I needed his help, he came through in a totally supportive human way that came as a real surprise. I felt that he could not have done it better.
>
> I was apprehensive yet clear when I went to tell him that I was going to resign from my full-time position, having invested ten years in what was a challenging and stressful job, latterly that of Business Group Manager. I explained that my wife's health had deteriorated and that I wanted and needed to spend more time with her and look after her as best I could. I also told him that I hoped that he would consider offering me a few days' work a month on a contract basis. This occasional work would be important in maintaining our financial stability.
>
> As we talked, I felt his immediate sympathy and care. He said that he believed that I was making the right decision and that, at a time like this, family needs have to come first; furthermore he would do his best to ensure that I had as much work as I was able to undertake. It also helped when he told me that he knew that my leaving the full-time payroll would be a big loss. I had really wondered if the company had rated me that much. He followed this up by writing to my wife telling her how much I would be missed and reassuring her that the company would support me to obtain part-time assignments so that she need not worry about our family finances.
>
> It has been two years since this conversation. I was able to be with my wife increasingly when she needed me and to spend some quality time with her when she was not feeling so ill, until she passed away some months later. I continued to work on an occasional basis through this period and to make ends meet. Given the situation, we both helped each other and both derived some benefit as a result. It was a win–win, which resulted in renewed mutual trust, but it all started with his caring and flexible response to my situation.

INDUCTION AND TRAINING

Great and expensive efforts are often made to recruit and select the right person for a job, only for them to be sabotaged by poor or even non-existent induction. It is an effective way of quickly demoralising and deskilling a potentially good recruit. This incompetence in induction is not universal. There may, for example, be careful induction for senior staff but none for others, or the other way round. Some managers may be casual, others rigorous. The human resources department may ensure effective induction happens or not bother.

As part of induction, new staff need to be given information on what to do in the face of severe problems or a crisis at home that may impact on their work, and what kind of support they might receive and from whom. They also need to be clear about family or compassionate leave policy, and to have a copy or easy access to one.

> A large retailer trained all its welfare officers in counselling skills and active listening in relation to bereavement, so that they could conduct their meetings sensitively with the next-of-kin of staff or retired staff who had died, and also make good judgements about follow up and/or referral. Another prominent media company, without welfare staff, trained its human resource managers in the same way for the same reasons.

One way or another, managers, supervisors, team leaders and staff representatives need to have:

- information and understanding of the bereavement process, and how it may affect staff;
- training in how to help affected staff, and how to find further resources that they may be able to draw on, within and outside the organisation.

AN IN-SERVICE STAFF SUPPORT NETWORK

Whilst some companies offer no additional support to that provided by managers, occupational health and the human resources department, many others provide more than that. Some, for example, have a cadre of volunteer supporters for staff under stress, such as bullying or bereavement, as an alternative or even in addition to an external counselling resource. One chemical company with whom I worked deliberately recruited an interesting cross-section of volunteers, including a shop-floor worker, a shop steward, a financial assistant, a director, a middle manager and a scientist from research and development. Their names, photographs and contact details were publicised in the hope that anyone in the company would feel comfortable talking to one or two people on the list. Some staff chose someone close to them in the organisation, while others seemed to go for someone more different or distant.

Other organisations have links to an external counselling resource, which may be in the form of locally based counsellors or through a contract with an employee assistance programme. This normally gives access to a 24-hour telephone helpline staffed by trained counsellors, perhaps some lawyers too, and also an option of face-to-face counselling sessions when wanted.

In addition or instead, some companies involve chaplains on a part- or full-time basis to provide emotional and spiritual support. In the USA, the demand has given rise to rent-a-chaplain firms such as Marketplace

Ministries or Corporate Chaplains of America. Because chaplains are on-site, employees can build relationships with them, so that there is less difficulty for some to access them when they feel that they need help.[18]

BEREAVEMENT COUNSELLING

People who can undertake bereavement support in-house should be identified, trained and briefed. A list of locally available external resources should also be compiled and publicised in the workplace. Bereavement counselling is described more fully in Chapter 4 and Appendix 4 lists some relevant national UK organisations in the field.

Those who have suffered a traumatic death and bereavement, for example, as a survivor of a fatal road traffic accident, may need debriefing quickly, but bereavement counselling is not relevant in many cases, particularly in the early days, especially if people are well supported within the community. That community may include the workplace, as well as the extended family.

> Some general practitioners, feeling no doubt under pressure themselves, started to refer all their bereaved patients immediately to the local branch of a bereavement charity. The branch chair of counselling explained to them that bereavement counselling was often not needed by many of those who are bereaved, particularly in the early few weeks. It was more appropriate for those people who had had exceptionally difficult bereavements, were especially isolated or felt stuck after a period of time: counselling can help in picking up and addressing the unfinished business left over from community support.

As someone who has both received and provided bereavement counselling, I know how valuable it can be, but it must not be pushed excessively. To do so can undermine the confidence and will of colleagues, family and friends to provide the kind of support that is crucial when we are bereaved.

Notes

1 Moores, R. (1994) *Managing For High Performance*, London: The Industrial Society (now the Work Foundation).
2 O'Donoghue, J. (1997) *Anam Cara: Spiritual Wisdom in the Celtic World*, London: Bantam Books.
3 Ryan, K.D. and Oestreich, D.K. (1991) *Driving Fear out of the Workplace*, San Francisco, CA: Jossey-Bass.
4 Wetton, L. (2003) *A Study into 'The Individual and Organisational Responses to Coping with Bereavement in the Workplace'*, Southampton: Southampton Institute.
5 Shellenberger, S. (1998) 'Workplaces can be tough on grieving employees', *Wall Street Journal*, 13 January.
6 Adams, A. (1992) *Bullying at Work*, London: Virago.
7 Shellenberger, S. (2000) 'Respecting bereavement needs (employee need)', *Association Management*, vol 52, no 9, September.

8 Management Best Practice (2002) *Survey: Managing Special Leave*, No 94, May, London: The Work Foundation.
9 Wetton, L. *ibid.*
10 Management Factsheets (2004) *Compassionate Leave*, March, London: The Work Foundation.
11 Tahmincioglu, E. (2004) 'Coping in grief, beyond "business as usual"', *The New York Times*, 1 February.
12 Trades Union Congress (1994) *A TUC Guide, Family Leave*, London: Trades Union Congress.
13 Stewart, A. (2003) *Playing For Keeps*, London: BBC Books.
14 Holmes, R. (2002) *The Last Taboo?* London: The Work Foundation, the gist.
15 Sting (2000) 'The 20th anniversary of John Lennon's death', *The Observer*, 3 December.
16 Ironside, V. (2004) 'Just give me a break', *The Times*, 3 April.
17 Trades Union Congress (1991) *A TUC Charter for Carers*, London: Trades Union Congress.
18 Eidam, M. (2004) 'Got worries? Tell them to the chaplain', *BusinessWeek*, 9 February.

Chapter 14

How people in different roles at work can help

- Company bereavement adviser(s)
- The human resources or personnel manager
- The line manager, team leader or supervisor
- The shop steward or staff representative
- The colleague
- The work group
- Teams as families?

In this chapter some of the different roles in an organisation that may have a particular part to play in providing effective support at a critical time are considered.

While some grieve mostly away from work and many find relief from getting on with the job, most people need to have their loss acknowledged with the opportunity for more active support being there from some people in the workplace.

> On the day after Christmas in 2002, Angelica Berrie, then the senior vice president for strategic planning at Russ Berrie & Company Inc., sat in the boardroom while directors discussed the future of the company. She was in a fog, she recalled. Russ Berrie, the company's founder and her husband, had died of a heart attack the previous day, and the executive committee had gone directly to work to choose a successor. . . . Ms Lewis took six months to grieve after her husband died. "I was on automatic pilot. I could not deal with anything. I was totally devastated." She advised others to "grieve, grieve, grieve".[1]

COMPANY BEREAVEMENT ADVISER(S)

It is helpful if someone in the organisation is identified as a focal point for good information about bereavement. If they have not already had it, some introductory training in active listening, counselling skills and the bereavement process will help them in this. They can coordinate and monitor the work of any internal or external network of people offering staff support for those who are bereaved or terminally ill, additional to support they are hopefully receiving from people in other roles considered in this chapter. In addition they need to maintain up-to-date information, local and national, on support and training resources in this area of work. This book can form part of that.

In large organisations and those with scattered sites, there may need to be someone local to that site with this role, supported and monitored by the person who acts as the company focal point.

These people can come from a variety of roles: human resources or personnel, occupational health, welfare or line management. People in each of these groups may aspire to be competent in bereavement support and many are, but equally they are likely to have wide-ranging remits. So it is not realistic to expect every human resources or occupational health person, for example, to be a specialist in this subject.

The role does not have to be occupied permanently. It can work well if it is passed on every three or four years – thus spreading the knowledge accumulated – so long as there is a careful handover. In recruiting and selecting such a person, their outside experience may be relevant. A line manager, for example, who is a volunteer counsellor or a Samaritan in their spare time, may be a good person to take on the role, although in other cases it will fit comfortably into an established human resources, occupational health or welfare department.

A critical element in the role of the adviser is to support line managers at all levels who are in turn supporting staff. Of course managers may seek help from any number of other people, such as their own senior manager, personnel manager, a colleague or an employee assistance programme. Whoever it is, they may really benefit from (and perhaps need to have) access to someone experienced on a confidential basis. They might consult, for example, about what they are finding difficult, the kind of support they are (and are not) offering, how the bereaved person seems to be or to off-load emotionally. The person consulted will need to find the right balance for both the bereaved member of staff and the manager by either:

■   supporting the manager to continue to provide support directly, or to see some other help inside or outside the organisation;

or:

■   a judicious mixture of the two.

Those familiar with the work of Macmillan and 'hospice at home' nurses will know that they can provide particular specialist support to people who are terminally ill and their families when they are at home. Help will also be available from others, notably district nurses. The latter can have a more or less collaborative attitude to the former. There are some parallels between their relationship and that of the bereavement adviser at work with the generalist human resources, occupational health and welfare person. There needs to be sensitivity, goodwill and mutual respect for such relationships to work properly.

THE HUMAN RESOURCES OR PERSONNEL MANAGER

Whether or not they are bereavement advisers or experienced in bereavement support, human resources or personnel managers may at any time be consulted about a bereavement, if only to clarify the compassionate leave entitlement.

> Tim, an insurance departmental manager, was helping one of his staff wrestle with a complicated claim, when the phone rang. It was Andrew's father: he would not be coming in that day. When the reason was explained, Tim forgot about the insurance query. A car had hit Andrew's wife and their six-month-old baby en route to the child minder: both had died. He managed to say that Andrew should take all the time he needed and for his dad to let him know if there was anything the company could do to help. When he put the phone down, Judy asked him what had happened. So he told her; at least that sorted out the problem of telling the staff. But what next?
>
> For the next half-hour Tim thought of nothing else. He remembered Andrew's pleasure when his son was born; the way he used to muck about, not least when playing football with some of the others during the lunch hour. His own daughter was about Andrew's age and their first grandchild was a few weeks older than Andrew's baby. He rang Emma in the HR division to tell her. She asked him if he wanted any help but he said that it was fine. Feeling claustrophobic, Tim got out of his office into the open plan area where his team worked. The atmosphere was not reassuring: uncannily quiet but not a lot of work seemed to be getting done. He realised what a close-knit group they were, despite or maybe because of the badinage and squabbling. The rest of the day was very strange. He didn't think that anything in particular was required of him, yet felt out of his depth. The next day, he rang Emma back: it might be useful to have a chat after all. So what does she need to think about as she prepares to meet up with him?

It is hopefully line managers who are the front line of workplace support to bereaved or terminally ill staff. The human resources manager's primary task is to ensure that they are adequately backed up especially in two ways: personal support and the provision of necessary information. They need to concentrate on their listening skills, in finding out how the line manager is feeling and also to help him or her sort out what issues need to be addressed.

Some managers feel safer in the first instance concentrating on the practical aspects, like compassionate leave and what the company should be doing. Having done that thoroughly, the manager may need to off-load some of what they are finding particularly difficult. That may include being deeply upset but imagining that they need to be 'strong' for the staff, to keep the ship afloat. Or they may feel guilty that they are not feeling very upset. Or they may be uncertain how far they should let the staff be distracted from their work and how soon they need to get things 'back to normal'. They are also likely to need affirmation and encouragement for what they are doing well in what could be unknown territory outside their skill base. On the other hand, they may have had experience of bereavement and be thinking that they know what the staff member is going through. Experience of bereavement can give a sense of what other people *might* be experiencing, but no one is an expert on another person's grief through their own experience. The closer the situations are superficially, the greater the danger of thinking that the inner experiences are the same.

The quality of the human resources manager's listening to the line manager needs to reflect the kind of listening the latter needs to offer the staff involved. Their ability to cope with the expression of raw grief (tears, rage, worry, guilt and panic) may be a factor in deciding who does what. Where the balance of direct support comes from will need to be worked out between the line manager and the human resources manager initially in the light of their workloads, availability, motivation and experience. The two of them will need to work out an agenda, a list of issues, that they need to consider and which will underpin their work together. It could look like this:

- the bereaved member of staff and the implications of the loss;
- time off and compassionate leave?
- funeral and practical short-term issues;
- return to work;
- immediate support;
- longer-term monitoring and support;
- the work group.

No death should be minimised, even though they are not all as obviously tragic as the one in the situation described above. An apparently routine death can be a cause of continuing disorientation, distraction and detachment from previous priorities at work. It is dangerous to make assumptions about what a bereaved person may be feeling and what their needs are. What is clear, however, is that the company needs to be seen to care about the bereaved member of staff and be assessing what their needs might be – and how far it is appropriate, desirable or possible for them to be met in-company.

Some managers find it helpful to have some relevant background reading about bereavement as well as organisations offering external support. Planning frequent contact in the early days with the line and/or HR manager is vital, beyond helping sort out the details of time off.

What other support, if any, the company should be giving and from whom also needs to be teased out. The level of support available from family, friends and others outside the company needs to be ascertained in case it needs supplementing at some stage. This may come from an external agency, such as CRUSE, or from the company. The latter may be supplied through self-referral to an employee assistance programme, an in-house counsellor or member of human resources or occupational health with relevant experience and training, if any of these exist. The company may also decide to bring in some specialist help from outside.

Bereavement counselling helps some but is not relevant to everyone who is bereaved. It should not usually be the first port of call, as the need for it often emerges some months or even longer after a death, if and when the bereaved person feels stuck and immediate support is drying up.

THE LINE MANAGER, TEAM LEADER OR SUPERVISOR

Good line managers, team leaders or supervisors want to take some responsibility for supporting bereaved staff out of their common humanity and personal ethics but it also makes sense in terms of their commitment to the task and productivity. Bereavement is a process that takes time, naturally and inevitably. It uses a great deal of emotional (and even physical) energy, some of which would otherwise be available for work.

If bereaved staff are supported through the process as well as possible, they are less likely to be alienated from their colleagues and the organisation and generally demotivated. The aim is to help them recover their ability to function positively in their life, including work, as soon as possible, without hurrying them artificially through the process. This is in their interests as well as that of the company. It requires, however, real patience. Time is likely to pass much more slowly for those grieving deeply than for those who work with them or around them, especially if there is an element of the impatient 'hurry bug' in the latter as there often is inevitably at work.

People managers need a 'whole-person' approach at the best of times, but certainly in times of bereavement. Each of us has one brain in one body, which is always with us! Our energy and attention are used on the task in hand, at work or at home. We may attempt to erect mental barriers between our professional and personal lives in order to switch off from one and concentrate more on the other. But the whole person, the whole of us, is always there. So it is no good imagining that bereavement and work motivation can always be kept disconnected.

Managers, therefore, need to ensure that they know about a bereavement in order to:

(a) communicate concern and support, both personally and on behalf of the company;

(b) ensure that the company, including managers and colleagues, are behaving in a supportive and appropriate manner, and are encouraged and, if appropriate, helped to do so;

(c) talk with the bereaved member of staff about their return to work and how they want to be supported after their return;

(d) ensure that the individual is being as well supported as possible, being neither isolated nor swamped.

The need for flexibility about agreeing or even offering compassionate leave is argued elsewhere. In the case of terminal illness, such leave may be as important before a person dies as afterwards. It often makes for a better relationship with the employer if such leave is granted properly, rather than the bereaved staff member having to go for a sick note. The general practitioner can, however, be very helpful to some people in working out when to go back to work.

In some situations the line managers need to provide direct support, but in others much less personally, so long as they are satisfied that adequate support is coming from someone. It will depend on:

- the needs and wishes of the bereaved staff member;
- the level of support being offered (and accepted) both in and outside work;
- the interest and competence of the manager in this area;
- counselling available in or through the company if required.

Although there are dangers of affirming the bereaved in such a way that communicates the message that what is valued is not showing grief, there is often a legitimate way of doing this. In describing the affiliative style of leadership, Daniel Goleman wrote about Joe Torre, '. . . the heart and soul of the New York Yankees. During the 1999 season Torre tended ably to the psyches of his players as they endured the emotional pressure cooker of a pennant race. All season long, he made a special point to praise Scott Brosius, whose father had died during the season, for staying committed even as he mourned. At the celebration party after the team's final game, Torre specifically sought out right fielder Paul O'Neill. Although he had heard the news of his father's death that morning, O'Neill chose to play in the decisive game – and he burst into tears the moment it ended. Torre made a point of acknowledging O'Neill's personal struggle and called him a "warrior"'.[2] There is a real sense of a coach here enabling and supporting players to grieve and appreciating that their love and commitment to their fathers is as completely and naturally compatible with their commitment to their team.

In situations where the staff member is off work to care for someone who is terminally ill, some contact can sometimes make a big difference, at least when the working relationship is good. Annie Hargrave, a counsellor, stopped working with people in the overseas emergency, aid and development business in order to care for her 21-year-old son when he was diagnosed with an incurable form of cancer in July 2001. She wrote subsequently, 'My supervisor, professional colleagues and the British Association for Counselling and Psychotherapy (BACP) were all very supportive, keeping alive for me that I was a working therapist, not currently at work. This phraseology helped me to maintain a good idea of this aspect of myself amidst the turmoil of what was happening. I found it much better than something like, "unfit to work", or "on indefinite leave of absence". Occasional meetings with my supervisor also kept alive the reality of the relationship between us'.[3]

'How is it going' meetings after the return to work are usually best at the end of the shift or the day, so that if the person becomes upset, they do not need to go back into work. The manager should not force them to talk in any depth if they do not wish to, but equally should make it clear that it is fine to talk about what they are finding most difficult at or outside work. The concern needs to be genuine and uninterrupted time should be spent with the bereaved member of staff, initially perhaps daily, even if only for a few minutes.

It is also important that support is not withdrawn suddenly, as if the bereaved are expected to shake out of their grief after a prescribed time, having used up their quota of care. The regular or ad hoc meetings with the line manager to see how things are going can become gradually less frequent. They are a means of monitoring how the member of staff is doing, especially but not only at work. These meetings can be quite low key. For some, it is good to interweave them with work discussions.

THE SHOP STEWARD OR STAFF REPRESENTATIVE

The trades unions have had a tough time in Britain in the past 25 years, but if they did not exist they would need to be invented. Many who have been indifferent to their existence find that they feel the need for them if they become the victim of what they consider to be unfair, perhaps tyrannical management behaviour. Suddenly a staff member can feel and be terribly powerless: the vulnerability of staff is the key to the importance of trades unions.

One stereotype of the trades union representative is that of a tough cookie spoiling for a fight with the management under any pretext, but the reality tends to be different. Many who agree to be put forward for election are people with both a desire for justice and also a genuine wish to be of help to other people, especially, of course, those they represent. Bereavement or serious illness are good examples of that vulnerability. The staff concerned may naturally talk to their shop steward, whose support is unlikely to be restricted to negotiating how they are to be treated by management. Indeed such negotiation may not even be required. But some representatives can still provide great support directly to the staff member and also influence colleagues in a positive direction.

Paul, one of Andy's team, died horribly in a forklift truck accident in the warehouse, and it was Andy who found him, still alive just but very severely injured. There was a horrendous half-hour before Paul was finally removed and taken to hospital, although he was dead on arrival. Andy's manager was, though well meaning, weak, emotionally pretty illiterate and generally of no help. The company's human resources manager saw counselling as a waste of time and probably likely to make things worse, and ignored Andy, other than to pressurise him to complete the accident procedure fast and cooperate fully in the ensuing investigation. It was his shop steward who took Andy on one side, provided some personal support and encouraged him to go at least to see his family doctor. This led to some short-term counselling at the surgery. In Andy's case, this made a huge difference in enabling him to cope and exercise leadership and support in helping the rest of the team come through the experience, both at work and at the funeral. It also helped him to relate to Paul's widow genuinely, something that he felt would be impossible in the immediate aftermath of the accident.

The listening and pastoral skills needed by staff representatives are acknowledged where they are included in shop steward, convenor and other training courses.

THE COLLEAGUE

The survivor of bereavement is 'catapulted', as Carol Staudacher has put it,[4] 'into a morass of responsibilities, requests for decisions, paperwork, and a stream of tedious, confusing, and often time-consuming details'. Some of this activity can be a way of occupying the mind so that the bereaved person is doing something practical in relation to their bereavement, while being distracted and protected temporarily from some of the painful feelings. Activity can help get the person through the worst of the early days. On the other hand, the pressure to do anything can also be incredibly hard for the person in the grip of acute grief (see Chapter 2). So, offers 'to pitch in', either by doing things or supporting the bereaved person to do things, can be a very real help especially, but not only if their family support is very limited. Examples could include any or all of the following:

- Make preliminary contact with a priest, minister, rabbi, the British Humanist Association or other spiritual representative.
- Contact a funeral director.
- Contact relatives and/or friends who need to be notified.
- Contact the line manager or personnel/HR department and/or colleagues, and pass on instructions about what should be communicated to others at work.
- Accompanying him or her to register the death.
- Prepare and deliver a notice for the newspaper.

- Prepare and despatch invitations to the funeral, if appropriate.
- Help decide on flowers or donations (and if so, to what).
- Provide and/or organise accommodation for visitors to the funeral coming from further afield.
- Accompany the bereaved person to visit the hospital mortuary or the undertakers to view the body.

These possibilities, perhaps supported by one of the checklists in Appendix 1 at the end of the book may be a useful basis for discussion with a bereaved colleague or at least to guide your own support for them.

THE WORK GROUP

Even though the feelings of anguish can be powerful in many workplace situations where a working group is disrupted, in a separation through death, however, it is likely to be particularly intense. Its finality is so powerful. When a colleague was killed suddenly in a road crash, his empty desk was a constant reminder. After a few days someone was brought in as cover and that felt almost shocking to see a replacement so soon, as if his memory was not being honoured, even though in practical terms the work needed to be covered. There are parallels here with the timing of bringing a new hospital patient into a bed or bed space previously occupied by someone who died on the ward. Much of this book deals with the need for management to attend with care and sensitivity to the needs of a bereaved work group.

The death of someone who left some time before to go to another job or retire is, however, less immediate. In such cases, the work group is likely to have re-formed. Colleagues may as a consequence miss the grieving of others, because if it exists it may be more unspoken. Yet the death of a retired colleague may be a source of acute sadness to those with whom a close relationship had been built, even if the group as a whole is also less affected.

TEAMS AS FAMILIES?

Teams or other work groups have something in common with families. Relationships can be more or less close or distant, depending on a variety of circumstances, including geography and the degree of trust that they generate. At best they provide familiar support structures that allow people to venture out into the world beyond the team and take risks and grow, knowing that there is always a consistent base to return to. Or they can feel claustrophobic and unsafe, inspiring the need to escape.

Traditionally at least one or two people are seen as head of the family, who can be relied on to protect and take the lead in decision making, although the baton of responsibility may be passed from one person to another for various reasons. Within the team, alliances form that may split its coherence at times. For this and other reasons, teams always struggle with becoming or avoiding being dysfunctional. This results in problems and misery for the people involved and outsiders who come into contact with the team may well pick up the bad vibrations.

When bereavement occurs within a team, as in a family, the following effects may be noticed and experienced:

1. A previously strong structure is rocked, pushed or shaken into a different shape.
2. Sometimes some people behave in unexpected ways for good or ill.
3. Emotions are running high and arguments may increase.
4. Hidden conflicts and feelings may reveal themselves. The bereavement may act as a catalyst. Secrets – the undiscussables – may come spilling out unexpectedly.
5. New responsibilities may need to be taken on by team members who perhaps shouldered little before, and who may rise to the challenge.

   In an already dysfunctional team, the danger is that existing problems are often made worse by the bereavement, sometimes providing the last straw to cause rifts and chasms so that they need a great deal of extra support from outside. On the other hand, bereavement may help team members to put into perspective and to one side some of their previous moans, grievances and personality clashes. Being part of a working group can enable mutual support to be undertaken naturally and in such a way that strengthens it. The team is then able to realign itself in its roles and functions to be able to cope with its future. The team leadership may need to be proactive in some or all of this, but equally there is likely to be a significant place for a light hand on the tiller, allowing members to have the oxygen to breathe deeply and take their own initiatives.

Notes

1 Tahmincioglu, E. (2004) 'Coping in grief, beyond "business as usual"', *The New York Times*, 1 February.
2 Goleman, D. (2000) *Leadership That Gets Results*, Harvard, MA: Harvard Business Review.
3 Hargrave, A. (2003) *Fit to Work*, Rugby: BACP in Counselling and Psychotherapy Journal, March.
4 Staudacher, C. (1991) *Men and Grief*, Oakland, CA: New Harbinger Publications.

Chapter 15

Helping the bereaved person at work

■ Parallels between bereavement and preparing for death
■ The terminally ill member of staff
■ When someone dies
■ Reticence and openness at work
■ Am I going mad?
■ Repetition and time-scales
■ Viewing the body
■ The funeral
■ Returning to work after someone has died
■ What not to say and what to say
■ The 'cross over to the other side' response
■ Practical help
■ Solidarity with the bereaved
■ Taking care of yourself

In this chapter, how to help those at work passing through the stages of bereavement is considered further. Much of this has some relevance for someone facing their own death reasonably imminently, whether or not they are still working, which is explored in more depth in Chapter 7. There may be as many as three phases:

1. When someone is dying.
2. When someone dies.
3. After someone has died.

All three situations can be highly charged emotionally. People act and react differently, but often with powerful feelings, whether or not they show them at work. To be on the receiving end of the expression of a lot of distress does not necessarily mean that you have hurt the feelings of the other person or have made matters worse by your behaviour. They may well have already been upset: all you have hopefully done is given permission or stimulated them, perhaps unintentionally, to share how they feel. So long as your response is sensitive and respectful, they will hopefully feel supported. For the first of these situations 'when someone is dying', Chapters 6 and 7 are particularly relevant, but this chapter concentrates on the issues facing a colleague who has been bereaved. Chapters 8 and 10 may also be relevant in their consideration of the practical tasks after someone has died and on funeral arrangements.

PARALLELS BETWEEN BEREAVEMENT AND PREPARING FOR DEATH

The process of bereavement overlaps with the stages of the emotional response to dying described in Chapter 7, Preparing for Dying and Death. A bereaved person who has supported someone in his or her journey towards death sometimes notices this, perhaps in retrospect. Indeed, the sharing of that sorrow can be a source of comfort to both the dying person and the one to be left behind and can give them both the sense that their love for each other on one level is stronger than death. For the survivor, however, the helplessness in their anticipatory grief can be agonising, as they come to realise that they are powerless to prevent the death of someone for whom they care so deeply.

THE TERMINALLY ILL MEMBER OF STAFF

The terminally ill person has two separate clusters of needs. One is the need for effective symptom relief and care (emotional and practical). The other is the need for time with friends and loved ones while there is still the opportunity. Line managers should regard it as one of their responsibilities to check out whether these needs are being met once the nature of their situation is understood. If the manager is not sure but suspects someone may be seriously ill, because of how the person looks or has been behaving or because of gossip, he or she needs to think both about whether to check it out and, equally important, how to do so. If in doubt, check it out, but do so with great care and discretion. Of course there may be another avenue via occupational health, although there may be confidentiality boundary issues there. It is often more straightforward to have direct communication. First of all, choose a time, perhaps at the end of the day or before a lunch break, when a sensitive conversation can be had without embarrassing the member of staff unnecessarily by them having to go straight back into work. Secondly, think through the level of support so that you can reassure genuinely and follow through with what you have said. Your aim should be that they feel relieved to have had the conversation with you, not have their worries stoked up. Then share your dilemma or ask a direct question, such as:

- I have been wanting to check out how you are but I did not want to seem intrusive.

- How are you, because you have seemed a bit weary (under the weather or whatever word is suitable) recently?
- I know you have not been well and wanted to check out how you are feeling now? I don't want you to overdo it here if that is going to make things worse (or get in the way of your recovery).

As far as quality time with others is concerned, it may not be helpful only to grant leave when there is a crisis: it can be very important to spend time together on good days too. This is where a flexible approach to leave entitlement by an enlightened line manager can be crucial.

The line manager needs to acknowledge the person's illness at regular intervals, however discreetly. To establish the current situation, open, non-threatening questions can be used, asked with discretion and care. In particular, the line manager will want to:

- stress that the company remains committed to the person concerned, and their family, if appropriate, as human beings and not just as units of production;
- reassure the person that the company understands and accepts that the person's work effectiveness is likely to be affected.

If powerful analgesics are being taken to control pain, it may be necessary to relieve the employee of certain tasks, such as those that require intense concentration, involve safety issues or are physically arduous. But managers and occupational health staff will need to exercise much tact to avoid creating a sense of uselessness. Colleagues will hopefully be willing to help out temporarily by taking on additional or alternative work, if they understand the reasons. There is a fine balance to be struck here between being open with them and respecting the staff member's desire for discretion and confidentiality. It is usually best to agree with him or her what it is appropriate to say, to whom and under what circumstances.

Periodic, informal discussions between manager and staff member can help in monitoring how things are going. Essential for such meetings will be:

- adequate time;
- a private setting, with comfortable chairs and a box of tissues available;
- the willingness to hear how things really are;
- the capacity to accept strong emotions (including tears) without embarrassment or anxiety;
- thoughtful timing: preferably before a meal break or going-home time.

The temptation in such a meeting to divert or interrupt tears or anger or to pretend that they do not exist, for example, needs to be avoided. The manager has to reach the point in their own development where they are either comfortable with the expression of strong feelings or at least can cope with them. It is important that they do not give out subtle or not so subtle messages that they want the person to become less emotional. Fleeing from or getting rid of the member of staff may be a way of acting this discomfort out:

> 'I will go and get you a glass of water/cup of coffee. . . .'
>
> 'Why don't you go and talk to personnel. . . .'
>
> 'Would you like to go to the ladies until you feel a bit better. . . .'
>
> 'Perhaps you would like me to leave you for a while until you feel a little better. . . .'

All of these responses give out the message that this is not the manager's business and is possibly wasting their time, although they are prepared to talk in a sensible way, if the member of staff can present their difficulties or problem in a coherent way. Whereas what the staff member may need is the opportunity to share their feelings and/or confusion. They might or might not then reach the point when they are able to articulate their needs.

The acceptance of how the person is feeling is often best communicated by a combination of active listening and reflecting the person's feelings back in your own words. For example, the manager might say: 'It feels very painful, George', or 'I can see how much you care about him'. The agenda for such a meeting will be to check out how things are both at work and at home, what the member of staff's current needs are and what, if anything, the company might do differently to help.

WHEN SOMEONE DIES

When someone dies, condolence and support need to be offered as soon as possible to the bereaved person, whether it is a staff member who has died or a partner, next-of-kin or another close relative or friend. Circumstances will help determine the best method – telephone, personal visit or letter. If in doubt, risk being more, rather than less, personal. But it may be the time to stand back a little, given that the crucial time for the company will be during the transition back to work (in the case of a bereaved person), and when the immediate family and friends are beginning to relinquish their close support.

It is important to find out early, however, whether the bereaved person does in fact have family and friends to provide support. If emigration, death, dementia or a family feud has removed them from their life, the organisation may be best placed to fill such a gap. Where employers have encouraged mobility, and therefore contributed indirectly to breaking up the extended family, it may be especially fitting if they make an early response.

If that is the case an appropriate person can, on behalf of the company, support them through the practical tasks that need doing, and in doing so sensitively, also provide emotional support in their grief. One of the check-lists in Appendix 1 may be helpful here, and possibly even for the member of staff, although beware: to give them a checklist at this stage can come across as too contrived and clinical in the wrong sense of that word.

As always, support needs to be person-centred. If the grieving person wants to be left largely alone, this should be respected. Some monitoring is advisable however, because, although a degree of privacy is natural in grief, too much isolation is rarely the best basis for mourning. It can lead to an intensity of grief that is too much, leading to, in exceptional circumstances breakdown or even suicide.

RETICENCE AND OPENNESS AT WORK

A useful way of looking at our own and other people's behaviour in a variety of situations is depicted in the Johari Window,[1] a well-known model highlighting four aspects of personality:

	Known to self	Unknown to self
Known to others	1. Open	2. Blind
Unknown to others	3. Hidden	4. Unknown

1. *Openness.* In this area, others and we know the impression we are giving.
2. Sometimes we are unaware and may have a *Blind* spot: we leak out information about attitudes, our thoughts and ourselves unintentionally and without awareness. Others may have a better idea of what we are thinking than we do.
3. At other times part of us is *Hidden*, in that we conceal our behaviour, thoughts or feelings from other people, perhaps deliberately.
4. We also have part of ourselves that is *Unknown* and deeply hidden, to ourselves and to others.

The principle of the Johari Window is that if we open ourselves to others, through self-disclosure, and allow others to show us more of ourselves, through feedback, the Open area is enlarged at the expense of all the other three areas. This can promote honesty and understanding, which in turn increases trust, all of which strengthen relationships in such a way that we are more likely to work together effectively, whether we are building a team, a family or a friendship.

Openness is, however, not always desirable. Taken to the extreme it can lead to an inappropriate 'letting it all hang out', which may result in us dominating situations with our own concerns, while others hardly have a chance to get a word in edgeways. It is sensible to assess with whom and in which situations openness is appropriate. Even then openness is for most people a matter of degree. Some people are very open to the point where they can come across as socially unskilled or insensitive.

In bereavement we may talk without discernment to too many people, too often at the wrong times and too publicly. At times this may be un-avoidable, if the power of our distress overwhelms us unexpectedly. A helpful colleague may respond flexibly and take us aside and give us a little time and support in order to share what is happening to us and then to recover enough to go back into a more public setting. We may be surprised that such an outburst can occur some time after the bereavement, triggered unexpectedly sometimes by the smallest thing, a chance remark or memory. Colin Parry wrote after the death of his 12-year-old son in the Warrington bombing: 'You must be prepared for many, many weeks during which odd little events will trigger off irrational responses. I remember almost breaking down in public when I heard a tune that Tim had loved. You will be shaken with grief when you see your lost child's look-alike playing in the street'.[2]

We are constantly deciding, in small as well as large ways, how much truth to share and how much time to take sharing it in any given situation. This is so natural a part of human interaction that it often happens without thinking. It is a healthy and normal inhibition, by which we protect our vulnerability while hopefully being sensitive to others. Reticence, therefore, has an honourable place in good relationships. But reticence too can be taken to an extreme: constant repression and evasiveness are as unhelpful as the opposite end of the spectrum. So we are looking for the right balance for any particular situation on the continuum between:

Repression/Suppression ⇔ Reticence ⇔ Openness ⇔ Let it all hang out!

Some people may appear to be evasive at work and not to want to talk about their bereavement, because it is too painful and they are anxious that they may become too emotional and even more distracted from their work than they are already. Or they may just assume, without checking it out or being told otherwise, that the death (and bereavement) taboos operate in their work culture. They may fear that they will be judged as incapable of handling pressure, if they appear overly affected by their bereavement, and therefore not ready for a promotion, a merit award or an important assignment. As we have already seen, the habitual inhibitions that lie behind reticence do not function reliably when newly bereaved. So the colleague may judge that they may not be able to control their emotions, if they allow the lid to come off, even a little. On the other hand, they may believe none of this but want to try to use work as a reprieve from grief by focusing on their job, knowing that at home their bereavement will be dominating their time and attention.

> Darren's baby had died tragically when only six months old. There was a great surge of sympathy for him after the event from the other staff in the insurance company claims office, not least from a couple of women also with young babies. Their sympathy began to wear thin, however, when after a couple of days back at work, he returned to his routine of having a football 'kick around' with some of the other lads during his lunch break. How could he if he really cared, they felt; but we often need to begin to normalise our life with breaks from our grief. This was a good way for Darren to do it, even though privately he was going through hell in a way some of his colleagues never realised.

The bereaved staff member of course may not be receiving much support at home. It may not be available because he or she may live on their own and be relatively isolated or they may live with a partner or other people, and still be relatively isolated. Bereavement can be one of many factors that apparently trigger the break up of a marriage or other relationship. One that is already rocky is one in which partners are often unwilling or incapable of offering each other support. Even in a good relationship, some find it hard to receive support. Colin Parry again: 'The first thing that the families of the dead must do is to feel for each other. You have to close ranks and make allowances for each other. You see, my wife and I learned that people do not grieve according to schedules and timetables. There are wild and irrational mood swings. There were times when I was overcome by grief and anger and she appeared calm and controlled. There were times when the raw emotion was hers, and I was numb and frozen.'[3]

The situation may be exacerbated by denial, which (as discussed in Chapter 2) is hopefully temporary. As a consequence, managers and colleagues need to respect reticence, by not pushing the person to talk when they do not want to, while making it clear that they are more than willing to listen, if at some point that might help. They need to show that they are interested because they care about how the person is doing. They want to know how they are, out of concern rather than prurient or gossipy curiosity.

AM I GOING MAD?

Because the feelings can be so strong and unfamiliar, people grieving deeply, especially for the first time, not infrequently feel that they are going mad. This can be reinforced through some of the dreams and nightmares that the bereaved experience.

While asleep, the mind continues to work through the bereavement process. Just as some of the feelings are unfamiliar and often extremely powerful when we are awake, so dreaming allows the mind to range free from the constraints of logic or consciousness into the further recesses of grief. An example came from Andrea, a young school teacher, who told me about a dream that she had after the death of her grandfather, to whom she had been very close:

> We were sitting around in the cottage, in the sitting room. Granddad couldn't speak or move because he was dead, and just sat there. Everyone else carried on as if he wasn't there. I was sitting opposite him, and I could communicate with him. I was the only one who could hear him. I told him I loved him. It felt as if it was just the two of us, so close – and that no one else mattered.

The person who successfully repressed the feelings of bereavement the first time it happened to them might experience a double dose the second time round. This can be particularly significant for bereaved adults who have previously suffered a major loss as a child. This is discussed further in Chapter 3, Children and Young People.

To learn from a colleague or friend that these feelings are normal can be reassuring: it will not protect the individual from their power or impact, but it helps to know that others have walked that road and perhaps understand a little. It can also be reassuring for the person to work out that they are probably not going 'mad', but rather experiencing a very powerful aspect of grief, which will in time most likely pass or become less overwhelming.

REPETITION AND TIME-SCALES

Acute grief is part of the ongoing task of mourning and can continue for months, sometimes years. Some people start to feel guilty even after a week if they have not 'got over it' and even more so if they're still acutely grieving after a month. It is better to anticipate the possibility of months spent in this phase, on and off: two years is not unusual, although it is impossible to generalise. It means that work concentration and motivation may continue to be affected, perhaps only intermittently, for quite a time. Allowance should be made for that. With a valued member of staff, it will be a good investment in terms of their longer-term contribution and motivation.

> Margaret's mother died on Thursday. The following Monday, she was greeted at work by a friend and colleague with a crisp smile and an equally bright, 'All right, then?'.

The bereaved frequently experience guilt or anxiety because they cannot pull themselves together and 'snap out of it'. They feel or are made to feel that they are boring and poor company, because of their continuing preoccupation with their loss. They may need to share repeatedly the story of what happened and to go over again and again what especially hurts. This involves talking, but also discharging feelings by crying, laughing and raging, sometimes one after the other, sometime together. That may need a colleague or friend or two with the commitment, patience and understanding of why this is important, and the listening skills to let them get on with it.

Every time the bereaved person goes through how their loved one died, or the row they had recently or the wonderful times they had together or whatever else may be particularly difficult, they are likely to be peeling off another layer of the pain. Although it may seem like repetition, it is never quite the same the second, third, fourth or fifth time. To understand that progress in healing comes through apparent repetition is crucial in supporting the bereaved. An experience of such magnitude often needs and demands quantity as well as quality of support. Although much of it will be resolved away from work, recovery from bereavement is not an area in which to expect quick results. Supporting people in bereavement is unlikely to be like a sprint. For the bereaved person it is more likely to feel like a marathon with the finishing line ever receding from view, however hard they try.

Compassion fatigue can easily affect those who initially offer more than they are able to sustain. So they feel the need to withdraw. This can mirror the desire of most bereaved people at work to focus on getting to grips with their job as soon as possible. This should not, however, be confused with the idea that they have necessarily 'got over it'. Long-term working relationships require an equally long-term balance between concentrating on the job and commitment to the well being of the person.

VIEWING THE BODY

One issue that some people unfamiliar with death struggle with is whether to see the body. What is done with the dead body varies greatly in different cultures but people also, irrespective of that, make individual decisions that reflect what they think is most appropriate. Except in parts of northern England and Ireland, it is less common now in Britain for the body to remain at home between death and the funeral. That custom enables family and friends to spend unhurried time with the body, adjusting to the new reality and taking their leave of it together or alone. A variation on that is for the coffin to be brought home for some hours, perhaps up to the day before the funeral, for the lid to be taken off to provide an opportunity for mourners to visit and to pay their respects. The coffin lid is removed during some funerals, and mourners are invited to view the body at some point in or at the end of the service. This helps to mark the farewell and the beginning of a new stage in which the person lives on, apart from the body, in the hearts and minds of family and friends.

Although the person is no longer in the body, we relate to each other in and through our bodies. It is false therefore to pretend that we should have no deep feelings towards a person's body, once that person is dead. Our experience of each other is inextricably interwoven with each other's bodies, which we can see, touch, smell and hear. Time spent with the body can help mourners at their own pace separate their love and attachment for the person from their body.

Whether or not to view the body is inevitably a personal decision, one many feel strongly about. Some have done so and wished they had not, because their final memory of the person is a distorted image of death, possibly made more difficult if they have been artificially made up and laid out in an alien environment. Virginia Ironside wrote about the death of her father: 'Then there was seeing my father in the Chapel of Rest and wondering what he would have thought of the extraordinary hair style the embalmers had given him'.[4]

On the other hand, for many people it is an important aspect of their mourning. The physical reality of death is not necessarily more distressing than the imagined reality. Except where there has been serious facial injury, being with the dead body can help in coming to terms with the reality of death and moving through the healing process of mourning. Comfort can be derived from being with a loved one's body laid out in their own bed, and allows people to say their farewells in the familiar surroundings of the loved one's own home. Additionally, if someone dies, suddenly for example, time is needed before the people closest to them are ready to let go of their body. That the body changes physically, so soon becoming pallid and cold, for many can make it easier for them to accept that the person is no longer in it; that also can take time. In Chapter 3, we consider this in relation to children and young people.

THE FUNERAL

Colleagues need to be informed of the death sensitively and in accordance with the wishes of the bereaved, so that they can contribute to the ground swell of support needed at such a critical time. Unless requested otherwise, attendance at the funeral should be encouraged: it can help friends in their mourning of someone they valued or cared about. The employer may want to be officially represented and a turnout of those who knew the deceased well can be very supportive to the family, so long as attendance is genuine and voluntary. There should also be a letter of condolence from a senior manager, preferably the most senior person in the organisation who knew the bereaved or deceased personally. Equally, the next of kin's wishes need to be taken into account, often ascertained at a home visit. That kind of awareness and sensitivity will also apply to the questions of wreaths, flowers, charitable donations and attendance at the post-funeral wake. In rare cases they will want as few people at the funeral as possible and that includes work colleagues. In Chapter 10, funerals and 'rites of passage' are considered in more detail.

RETURNING TO WORK AFTER SOMEONE HAS DIED

Some bereaved members of staff find it helpful to visit the workplace before they come back, if only to see the manager, and maybe have a chat with colleagues to break the ice. Coming back part time for the first week or two also works well for some, though not for others. Concentration may be considerably reduced in the early weeks. Where safety is an issue or tight deadlines or other stressful situations are unavoidable, ways of protecting the member of staff in the short term should be explored.

When a person returns to work after the death of a friend or relative, colleagues are often embarrassed about whether to say anything and, if so, what. In general, if you have any kind of personal relationship with the grieving person, find a way to acknowledge their loss openly and as quickly as possible. The quality of your relationship may be impaired if this does not happen. Somehow the loss, sadness or tragedy needs to be made explicit. It should not be undermined by cheery or lugubrious variations on the theme of 'look on the bright side', a form of denial.

The first reference to the grief should be as natural as possible. It need not be in a separate office but should be discreet; a warehouse, corridor, factory bench or open-plan office may be perfectly adequate, as long as the conversation is private.

WHAT NOT TO SAY AND WHAT TO SAY

When you do meet, what do you say? What is usually unhelpful is to say anything that minimises the loss: it is not for you to reassure or look on the bright side. Examples of such well-meaning but inappropriate greetings to bereaved members of staff on their return to work include:

I'm sorry he died, but . . .

- I believe that it was expected;
- it must have been a relief for him/for you;
- he had a good innings;
- it means you can start to look forward now;
- we all have to go sometime;
- I'm sure you can have another baby.

To 'reconnect' with the person, say something simple and genuine, which expresses, directly or indirectly, how you feel. More important than the words are your concern and compassion. These will be felt and will shine through, since people tend to be especially sensitive at such a time. Do not expect it to feel comfortable: your discomfort may be an indication that you are being genuine and not putting on an emotional mask. Examples of what you might say include:

- I'm so sorry about Helen.

- You've been in my thoughts a lot these last few days.
- Tom, I just don't know what to say.
- Tom, I can't find the words to tell you how sorry I am.
- He was a great person: it's a terrible loss.
- If you ever feel like talking, you know where I am.
- Why don't you bring the children over for a meal at the weekend?

All of these responses could jar if they are not from your heart, so they are given as examples only of the kind of phrases that can be authentic.

THE 'CROSS OVER TO THE OTHER SIDE' RESPONSE

The worst we can do for each other in these circumstances is metaphorically to cross over to the other side of the work street, allowing our embarrassment, indifference or mistaken sense of sensitivity to leave the bereaved alone. Suffering is seldom minimised by avoidance, although to go to the opposite extreme is also crass. Do not endlessly return to the subject, asking them how they are when they are engrossed in their work or in front of other people. Their discomfort may be increased, because the person concerned feels more isolated if they are singled out too conspicuously. This response is all too frequent and hurtful. A wise way of avoiding denial is to afford the bereaved a settling-in period (a few minutes or hours), and then actively seek the person out, rather than leaving an encounter to chance.

> On Bill's return to work after his mother's premature death, he found a note on his desk querying his time off. The personnel officer did not know about his bereavement, and subsequently apologised for what had happened. Nevertheless, Bill felt hurt and angry that he felt that he had to sort out with his line manager, on his first day back, a muddle over his compassionate leave.

PRACTICAL HELP

In some traditions, the extended family and neighbours take responsibility for all meal preparation for the bereaved during their first month of mourning (see Chapter 11). The offer of practical help as well as emotional support is always worth considering. It may not be needed, because others have stepped in. But it can still be an effective way of acknowledging what has happened, and may be really welcome and appreciated. If people feel able to accept such help, it is excellent to provide it, but, as always, make the offer but do not push it. Work colleagues will know more than they first realise about practical ways of helping: a meal left for their freezer, transport for children, partners and elderly dependants and tidying the garden before the funeral. It may also be helpful to offer to go with the person to register the death, and to help sort out any urgent financial matters or funeral arrangements.

What happens once the person has returned to work and the loss has been explicitly acknowledged? Some colleagues will breathe a sigh of relief that it is over and lapse into the 'ignore' mode. But, however well disguised it may be, grieving will continue long after the return to work. This may be uncomfortable to be near: another person's loss can remind us of our own past griefs as well as our human vulnerability and mortality.

SOLIDARITY WITH THE BEREAVED

On a day-to-day basis, we may live as if death is not part of our personal reality. That illusion is undermined when death gets uncomfortably close to us. If we want good human relationships, we have to live with our discomfort and acknowledge our solidarity with the bereaved. Practically, this will involve action such as:

- periodically ask how they are;
- continue to be prepared to make time for them;
- offer attentive listening;
- give them 'permission' to talk or not talk;
- review what practical support might be appropriate as time passes.

TAKING CARE OF YOURSELF

Bereavement puts demands on our physical, mental and emotional resources, so it is important that extra care is taken at such a time. It is easy to forget or neglect to do this in the midst of all that is going on. The following are examples of what the bereaved person can do to take care of themselves:

- Drink plenty of water;
- Eat regular nutritious meals, with plenty of fruit and vegetables;
- Ensure that you have regular exercise, as enjoyable as possible, preferably some of it in the fresh air;
- Breathe deeply and easily, filling and emptying your lungs fully;
- Beware of increasing your intake of coffee, tea, alcoholic drinks, cigarettes, sweets or junk food: consider cutting back to avoid getting more depressed through that avenue;
- Be prepared to allow time and the opportunity to talk through what happened and its impact on you with those close to you, if they are able and prepared to listen, and/or with someone in a counselling role;
- Give yourself the best chance of sleeping well, but if you cannot, be prepared to get up and do something else before trying again;
- Relax to reduce muscle tension through some combination, for example, of meditation, swimming, relaxation exercises, walking, soaking in a hot bath and massage.[5]

The need for taking care of yourself after a bereavement and also for taking notice and supporting others who experience that kind of loss is illustrated by the scoring of it in 'The Life Change Index'. This is taken from *Strategies in Self-Awareness*, published by The Marylebone Health Centre bases in London[5] and reproduced as the addendum to this chapter.

Notes

1   Luft, J. and Ingham, H. (1995) *The Johari Window: A Graphic Model of Human Relations*, California, LA: Extension Office, Western Training Laboratory in Group Development, University of California.
2   Parry, C. (1998) 'Grief, anger, yes. But don't be poisoned by hatred', *Daily Mail*, 17 August.
3   Parry, C. (1998), *ibid.*
4   Ironside, V. (1992) 'On a voyage without my father', *The Times*, 29 July.
5   Holmes, T.H. and Rahe, R. *Life Change Index* in Strategies in Self-Awareness, London, The Marylebone Health Centre.

Table I The ranking of 43 common experiences on a numerical scale of Life Change Units (LCU), after Thomas H. Holmes and Richard Rahe

Rank	Life event	LCU value	Rank	Life events	LCU value
1.	**Death of a partner**	100	22.	Changes of responsibilities at work	29
2.	Divorce	73	23.	Son or daughter leaves home	29
3.	Separation	65	24.	In-law trouble	29
4.	Spell in jail	63	25.	Outstanding personal achievement	28
5.	**Death of a close family member**	63	26.	Partner starts/stops work	26
			27.	Begin or end school	26
6.	Personal injury/illness	53	28.	Change of living conditions	25
7.	Marriage	50	29.	Change of personal habits	24
8.	Loss of job	47	30.	Trouble with employer	23
9.	Marital reconciliation	45	31.	Change in working hours or conditions	20
10.	Retirement	45			
			32.	Change in residence	20
11.	Change in health of family member	44	33.	Change in schools	20
12.	Pregnancy	40	34.	Change in recreation	19
13.	Sex difficulties	39	35.	Change in church activities	19
14.	Gain new family member	39	36.	Change in social activities	19
15.	Business merger/change	39	37.	Smaller mortgage or loan	17
16.	Change in personal finances	38	38.	Change in sleeping habits	16
17.	**Death of a close friend**	37	39.	Change in number of family get-togethers	15
18.	Change to different type of work	36			
			40.	Change in eating habits	15
19.	Change in number of arguments with partner	35	41.	Holiday	13
20.	Having a large mortgage or loan	31	42.	Christmas	12
21.	Foreclosure of mortgage or loan	30	43.	Minor violations of the law	11

Notes
A score of over 300 points in one year is said to increase the risk of becoming ill in the following 2 years by 80%.
A score of between 150 and 300 points in one year is said to increase the risk of becoming ill in the following 2 years by 51%.

Chapter 16

Death at work

- When someone dies at work
- Accidents and murders
- Police statement-taking
- The organisation's response to a death at work
- The initial visit by the line manager
- Debriefing
- Responding to anger
- Support options
- Follow up by the line manager
- A follow-up period of one-to-one counselling
- Visits from senior management

WHEN SOMEONE DIES AT WORK

If someone dies at work, whether a colleague, customer or supplier, the event inevitably and rightly has a powerful impact. How that impact is managed is crucial to the way staff can cope. If it is handled badly, it can cause unnecessary longer-term difficulties for staff, quite apart from alienating them from a management they may perceive as inadequate, uncaring or both. If the person has committed suicide, the level of stress on those remaining is likely to be even greater. This is considered in particular in Chapter 9 'Suicide, stress and bullying'.

In some work settings, death is to be expected. Nevertheless, even in hospitals or a hospice, the death of a colleague or a friend can be devastating. The humanity of staff there is a crucial element in their ability to help others in their dying and bereavement. Their own vulnerability means that they are as much in need of support when they are directly bereaved as anyone. War is another extreme example of a workplace where death not only happens but killing is part of the job. Some members of the armed forces can be traumatised by what they have experienced or done themselves. The grief of a man or woman is likely to be more complex, though not necessarily more intense, over fellow human beings they have killed because they were temporarily assigned to the role of enemy than that of the death of a comrade. After the first Gulf War 1990–1991, research[1] indicated those American marines being treated for post traumatic stress disorder commonly suffered from the following symptoms:

Sleep disturbance   (41%)
Hyper-irritability   (38%)
Hyper-alertness   (36%)
Emotional numbing   (28%)
Intrusive thoughts or flashbacks   (23%)
Family or interpersonal problems (22%)

The stress of war is compounded by its extreme physical and psychological demands and moral ambiguity, as well as the experience and fear of being the victim, witness and perpetrator of deliberately inflicted suffering and death.

Members of the armed forces can share with nurses, doctors or members of the ambulance, fire or police services a struggle with guilt because they feel that they could have done more to prevent someone's death. Such guilt or regret is often an inevitable part of real care and commitment, even though the guilt has to be managed or worked through so that it does not become incapacitating.

A disaster may be on a small scale, although no less devastating in its impact, albeit on a small number of people, perhaps especially on an individual. Or it may be much larger, as in the case of a terrorist outrage or a natural disaster: earthquakes, fires, train crashes, raids, bombings, kidnappings or malicious attacks, which can all result in people dying or being very seriously injured.

Good employers need their own contingency plan, so that they know what to do if the worst happens. The plan needs to be formulated and followed through so that key people are clear about what is expected of them and sufficiently coached and trained, so that they can fulfil those expectations. Such a plan needs to include three core elements:

- the immediate support of staff, practical and emotional;
- debriefing by people trained appropriately;
- a follow-up period of voluntary one-to-one counselling over a period of three weeks in the first instance for those who might especially need it.

ACCIDENTS AND MURDERS

The words accident and incident are typically used to describe violent events, although the words often feel inadequate. Many crashes or collisions are the result of incompetent or selfish driving, even though they may be road traffic accidents. To talk of road traffic accidents can seem to undermine the responsibility for causing them, which can matter greatly to the victims or their relatives. Incident is a bland word, even though what happened may have been violent and traumatic. The phrase 'post-incident support' is used to describe the support needed for people who have been in a frightening or potentially frightening situation, often at work.[2]

Deaths resulting from 'accidents' and murders produce the agony of feeling that they were unnecessary, caused by human folly or wickedness. They happen to people irrespective of their health and age and, therefore, generate the strongest feelings among the survivors. Over 22,000 people have, for example, been killed at work as a result of accidents in the past 30 years in the UK.[3] If the employer is found to be grossly negligent, the Health and Safety Executive may recommend a prosecution for corporate manslaughter after its investigation, although this is rare. The British Crown Prosecution Service accepts such cases even more rarely. What is more frequent in the UK is a prosecution under health and safety legislation. The time taken by and the delays in these investigations themselves are an added source of stress. If all of this takes, for example, a year or more, the bereavement process can be slowed down. The bereaved can feel that they are being kept in a sort of limbo.

Calculated risks in economising with equipment and/or training have been estimated as a cause for about 60% of fatal so-called accidents at work.[4] The anger that people feel in bereavement is reinforced if the employing organisation is believed to have caused it, because they were incompetent or did not care enough about their people. For those who are left, there may be a strong desire for justice to be done. It may be fuelled in part by a desire for revenge but also by their commitment to the person whose life has been taken away. There is a need to make sense of their death and find some good in the evil, perhaps in helping to prevent such tragedies in future, so that the person may be thought of as not having died completely in vain.

> On 16 July 1990, 24-year-old John Leadbetter fell to his death down an unguarded shaft on a construction site in central London, nine months after the death of Brian Billington, who fell down another unguarded shaft on the same site. At the inquest, the jury returned a verdict of accidental death, leaving relatives devastated and furious, especially after the coroner reportedly refused to accept the possible relevance of the earlier accident. The Construction Safety Campaign has organised pickets in recent years outside inquests to raise media and public awareness of the issues.[5]

Survivors of 'accidents' or 'incidents' can be helped, in a bizarre kind of way, if they have a visible injury, so long as it can heal. It is like a badge, which others can see and acknowledge. On the other hand, if the injury is both facial and felt to be seriously disfiguring, this can bring in an extra dimension of distress. Guilt at apparently getting off lightly in a situation when others have died can cause guilt as well as relief, especially if the survivor saw or was with some of those who perished. Survivors with no injury, on the other hand, may feel traumatised but their psychological wounds are invisible to those without awareness or imagination.

POLICE STATEMENT-TAKING

If a statement is needed in the case of a death in suspicious circumstances, the police will generally want to take it as soon as possible after the incident, because facts and memories can so easily become distorted over time, not least with repeated telling. If the interview is carried out sensitively, it may not only help catch suspects but also reduce the level of trauma by providing some scope for emotional release. That, however, is not the main aim. The police must ask thorough and searching questions, which can in some instances come over as too challenging and critical. Some police officers are less emotionally competent than others, and the procedure can be upsetting. It may help to suggest that a colleague is with the member of staff during the interview, so that any necessary support can be provided during it and especially afterwards.

THE ORGANISATION'S RESPONSE TO A DEATH AT WORK

If someone dies in the course of work or duty, not only their family but also their immediate colleagues need to be informed carefully and quickly, so that they do not hear either through the grapevine or media first. Sometimes the latter is impossible to avoid, in which case it has to be accepted. With the speed of 24-hour communications through the media, it is a time for quick thinking and quick action by the company, buttressed by good media planning. For colleagues off sick or on holiday, equally careful consideration needs to be given to the appropriateness and feasibility of informing them while away from work.

Some general guidelines have been produced by Gary Mayhew[6] identifying useful points to consider in the event of a potentially traumatic event, some of which are useful in thinking about appropriate responses to a sudden death at work. These are listed below. Not all sudden deaths at work are sufficiently dramatic to attract media interest, in which case point 2 will be irrelevant:

1. Be aware of staff who have suffered other traumas; they may experience the old distress, compounded by the latest trauma.
2. Encourage staff to telephone home before the event becomes publicised through the media.
3. Inform absent staff of the event as this can spare them the shock of hearing about it from other sources or arriving at work without prior knowledge.

4. Ensure a coordinated, sensitive management response.
5. Expect short-term reduced efficiency from staff, including those who appear to be on the periphery.
6. Encourage (but do not compel) all staff to return to work the following day, even if they only perform light duties.
7. Arrange the debriefing, if possible, within 48 hours of the incident.

One Friday, Bob witnessed the death of a colleague at work some miles from their base. They had worked together for over a year. It took him an hour to summon help and get a doctor to the scene, who confirmed Jack's death. Bob helped get his body back to base, where his team leader found him sitting in a state of shock. The team leader checked that Bob had been with Jack, told him that he would have to answer questions in the investigation, but meanwhile to get back home and get some rest. Presumably this was well intentioned, but he never gave Bob a chance to say what happened or to talk about how he felt. He didn't know that Bob's parents, with whom he lived, had gone off on a week's holiday the day before. So Bob went back to an empty house and a long and lonely weekend, which he passed in a nightmarish state of confusion.

Twenty years later, Bob had been promoted to a job as a personnel manager, which on the whole he did excellently; but he found supporting staff after a bereavement or an accident exceptionally stressful. He sensed that in that area, he was considered to be a little inhuman and rigid, because he did not want to get into thinking about his own incident all those years before. He felt as if it had happened yesterday. A Counselling Skills course that Bob attended gave him more insight into how he had got stuck. It also provided an opportunity for him to talk through and to detoxify what had happened to him, as well as to Jack, so many years before.

Bob's team leader had, typically in those days, been given no briefing or training on how to support staff in such circumstances. Evidence is now emerging about what to expect after a traumatic event at work, especially if it is handled poorly. Staff may be distracted, demotivated and find it hard to work effectively or even to work at all. The latter may show up in levels of absenteeism and sickness. Incidents of alcohol or other drug-related problems might increase, along with interpersonal conflict and unpredictable disruption.

THE INITIAL VISIT BY THE LINE MANAGER

The immediate support of the staff is often best undertaken by a line manager, who would usually be the next most senior manager, who is not on leave, in the structure above the member of staff directly involved in the incident. Typically, good practice is for this to take place immediately or at least within 24 hours. As the company's representative, they need to communicate the message that they and the company are primarily concerned with their welfare. If there has been theft or physical damage to property, the manager has to communicate that that is a secondary consideration and may hardly mention it, at least on an initial visit. He will need to take on board staff concerns. That concern is primarily demonstrated by the quality of the manager's listening, through the way he asks what happened, how they are and how they feel.

Talking can help take the pressure off, hence the importance of the manager being prepared to listen as staff members tell him or her what happened in their own way. Check out what their worries and concerns are. Some of these the manager may be able to do something practical about in the short term, but it may be as important to show that the staff member has been heard accurately and with respect by acknowledging what they have said and how they feel. If staff are reassured too quickly, it can leave the impression that what they have said is being minimised and not taken seriously.

A well-intentioned remark meant to break the ice or the tension can easily backfire and be experienced as insensitive or uncaring if it is too light or even humorous. That is not to deny that humour might have a place, can be a helpful way of breaking the tension and sometimes has a place in coping with death. Thinking about the person who has died may include not only grief but also what they liked about them, and that may have an affectionate amusing tinge to it, but it usually comes later. Laughter is not, however, unknown in shock.

Managers demonstrate care or the lack of it through what they do or do not do, as well as the way that they do it: for example, organising transport home for staff who may be upset or in shock and not pushing people back to work immediately. If the police are involved, someone to provide support while statements are taken can also be helpful. While fitting with business needs, some people may need permission to take the time to recover in their own way. A little time out taken by staff in the short term is likely to result in normalising the situation more quickly in the longer run with their return to full motivation and productivity.

Lastly, the manager needs to be ready to give some information about their possible response, that for example it would not be surprising if they find themselves reacting strongly, once they are out of shock, two or three days after the incident. The information will be designed to help people know what to expect. What seem like abnormal responses in an abnormal situation may be very normal. The manager also needs to explain what will happen next, such as health and safety or police procedures, if relevant, and also what follow-up support both for the bereaved and for former colleagues will be forthcoming.

The importance of this initial support by the manager is reinforced in one company by making it a disciplinary offence for an area manager not to visit a branch within 24 hours of any raid, whether or not anyone was physically hurt, let alone killed.

In summary, the aims of the initial visit by the line manager are to:

- find out what happened;
- find out how people are by asking and listening well;
- ensure immediate help is offered and in place, if relevant, for the bereaved;
- check out communication to the bereaved, absent colleagues and, if appropriate, the media;
- offer and give information that may be useful;
- prepare staff for follow up, including the support that they and the company will provide for them.

For the manager to undertake this role effectively, a supportive and informed human resources manager, line manager or counsellor can, if there is time, assist and prepare for the visit and debrief after it – face to face or by telephone.

Peter Twist, a former senior officer in the Metropolitan Police, writes of an incident in a London police station, which he line managed at the time:

> Dave was a much-loved and respected police officer who had retired, after completing his service, to an administrative post in the Crime Support Unit of the sister police station where he had served for many years. Although he was still well known to his former colleagues, he was now particularly close to the other members of his office with whom he worked on a daily basis.
>
> His daily routine was to start work at about 7 a.m. and prepare for investigating the crimes reported overnight. This routine was dramatically interrupted when, at about 7.45 a.m., Dave became suddenly unwell and collapsed with what was, and gave all the appearances of being, a massive heart attack. Help from colleagues was quickly summoned and an ambulance immediately called.
>
> A male and female police officer, who had returned to the station after patrolling in a police car, gave first aid and the agitated wait for the ambulance began. After five minutes it was clear that Dave was dying and no satisfactory time of arrival of the ambulance could be ascertained. For better or for worse, the two officers decided to get Dave into their police car and drive straight to the nearest hospital.
>
> The frenzied dash to the hospital began, with one of the officers doing all she could in the rear seat to keep Dave alive. Sadly, all her efforts were unsuccessful, with the hospital casualty staff acknowledging defeat and pronouncing that Dave had been dead on arrival.
>
> Back at work, the majority of staff had started to arrive at 8.30 a.m. to be greeted by the dreadful news. Disbelief, shock and horror ran through the police station: rumours abounded and, into the middle of this vortex of emotions, the two exhausted and deeply shocked officers returned.

Dave's next of kin was the companion with whom he had been living since the break-up of his marriage and a woman well known to many of the staff. To inform her of the news, the two officers insisted on visiting her personally, a gesture which, though difficult for them, gave reciprocal comfort and a sense of reality to them all.

As the officer in charge of the police station, I naturally attended the office at once as soon as I was informed and spoke to all concerned. Returning to my office, I telephoned our Occupational Health Department and, within an hour, trained staff arrived and started an immediate debrief. Even at this early stage, their sensitive ears picked up the seeds of recrimination, criticism and misinformation and a formal debriefing session was arranged for all who wished to attend the following day.

This was invaluable in addressing the issues mentioned above and was especially appreciated by the two officers, who were able to give their colleagues a full and moving account of what they had done and why. In addition, care was taken to address the concerns of night duty staff.

Dave's funeral was held a week later and provided a significant tribute to and celebration of a lifetime of public service and companionship, unmarred by whispers of innuendo and condemnation.

Peter Twist spoke to the officers some time afterwards to see how they were doing in relation to the whole incident. The male officer appeared to have capably survived one more of the traumatic incidents, which had already peppered his career. His female colleague was reflective: 'I feel privileged to have been able to give what I hope was some assistance to a colleague in his dying moments'.

DEBRIEFING

A staff debriefing can be helpful if the death has been particularly upsetting for staff, especially for those who were there when it happened. It is designed to enable affected staff to share some of what they have experienced and are experiencing. This helps to normalise what they are going through, and to promote an environment of mutual understanding and support, in which they can talk (without being compelled) with each other about the incident and its aftermath, both for them as individuals and as a group. The debriefing operates at a factual and practical as well as at a 'feeling' level. It allows staff to discuss any worries about the incident, such as safety arrangements, first aid or response times. It will also be another chance to talk about future support options that are available.

Although the debrief may be undertaken effectively by a line or human resources manager, there are advantages of someone else experienced and trained in doing it, such as:

- possibly enabling people to speak freely, especially if the company response is thought to have been inadequate so far;
- demonstrating that the incident is being taken seriously;
- involving someone who may have something different to offer;
- enable any support subsequently given to the managers concerned to benefit from the added value of having spoken directly with the staff concerned;
- save some management time.

There are arguments on the other hand for doing it internally, either by a line manager or by a human resource or occupational health colleague with relevant skills in this area. Equally a specialist, external to the company, may also be a good choice, if the death has been traumatic for the staff who are left. It is important, if at all possible, not to start until the whole group is present. If someone can only be seen at home or in hospital, a visit needs to be made but limited to caring for the staff member rather than a full debriefing. An invitation can be made for that to take place at an appropriate later date.

A group debriefing is a combination of input and facilitating staff to listen to each other. The facts of what happened are the starting point; and then people's different perspectives on what happened and the impact on them in terms of how they have felt and have been since. The staff are encouraged to tell each other as well as the debriefer what has happened on a number of levels. They may have different views about what happened and also the impact it made and is making on them. Some or all of them may need to express their anger, guilt, fear or disappointment. To do that may make others feel less isolated, as they realise that they are not necessarily the only ones feeling the way they do. It is important that the debriefer does not respond defensively to anger, but allows it to be expressed.

Without such a debriefing, some staff may feel that everyone else is less affected than they are, which can become a source of resentment towards the others for not apparently really caring about the person who has died. The debrief is primarily a vehicle for staff support but the company may well learn something useful for future planning and management.

The input might include something about the normal responses and reactions to trauma, including some of the private symptoms, such as nightmares or seemingly irrational fears and anxieties that may worry some people greatly. These can lead to them assuming that they are signs that they are not 'hacking it' or coping, and be drawn into what could be unnecessary and premature decisions that they will have to leave. Staff need to be told that if they experience different, possibly even stronger, feelings at a later stage, not to be surprised. That is why it is good to keep an open mind about follow-up support, even if they feel it is not necessary now.

Lastly any suggestions made by those involved in the debriefing, as a group or by individuals, need to be seen to be taken seriously with a promise to think further about or to investigate their feasibility. Equally, promises in the heat of the emotion to make changes, which cannot subsequently be delivered, need to be avoided. Feedback is essential. Suggestions made at such a time, even if they are apparently small or even trivial, may carry the significance and emotional power of possibly preventing such a death in the future. They must not be treated lightly.

RESPONDING TO ANGER

A manager or any other company representative may be on the receiving end of some anger, which may feel justified or displaced. If the debriefing has been well done, safety will have been established for people to express how they really feel if they wish. Others may be in such a volatile state that they cannot control how they feel, even if they want to. Either way, the debriefer needs to receive the anger constructively. The following points may help:

- Relax yourself before the debriefing as far as is possible.
- Listen actively.
- Notice how people may be feeling with your eyes as well as your ears.
- Try to understand how they feel.
- Remember that the anger may be what is on top, but other feelings, such as fear, may lie below the surface.
- Acknowledge the anger you sense, using reflection.
- Remember that there is likely to be some truth, subjective if not objective, behind the anger, however irrationally expressed.
- Don't argue back or respond aggressively by raising your voice.
- Don't expect to resolve the problem there and then.
- Don't get fixated on the anger and ignore other feelings, which may be expressed, albeit less strongly.
- Reflect back what you are noticing, hearing and sensing.
- Be prepared to give it time, but go back to staff about issues raised at a later stage when some cooling off may have occurred.

SUPPORT OPTIONS

There are a number of different ways in which staff can seek the kind of support that they may require after a death at work. Some incidents are potentially rather than actually traumatic, in the sense that the same incident may stir up all kinds of stress for one person but for another it appears like water rolling off a duck's back. On the other hand, a member of staff who appears not to have been too deeply affected may react more strongly at a later stage.

Apart from counselling, some staff can be helped by relaxation (tapes or training), meditation, for example transcendental meditation, prayer, sport, swimming, running or massage as well as group discussion. It can be empowering to realise the variety of options that may help, none of them a panacea, but all likely to be better than excessive alcohol or other drugs in helping people recover from a traumatic experience. Some of these options many staff will use on their own initiative, or as part of their life outside work. Encouragement from management, however, to be open to the possibility of value being derived from some or all of these might help some staff get over the hurdle of embarrassment or resistance. Encouragement can vary from information, to 'Why not give it a go', to offering some time off, to providing it from within the company. It can also be useful to ask them 'How is it going?'. If it really isn't working, whatever it is, there are times when it is good to give it up rather than dragging on out of a misplaced sense of obligation.

Whether staff are 'under the doctor' or not, after an incident, good support avoids over-medicalising the situation. A 'sickness' label can stick in such a way that recovery may be impaired. The notion of being a 'victim' has similar dangers.

> The staff were very agitated in the open-plan finance section, after the husband of one of the staff had killed their youngest child on his second birthday. A counsellor was asked to come in to run some short support sessions for staff in groups of about half a dozen, prior to the baby's mother returning to work. The departmental head told the counsellor that she was particularly concerned about Alec, one of the supervisors and a young father himself who had attempted suicide two months previously after a row with his partner. In the event, Alec told the counsellor that he had just been to hell and back and was not intending to have a return visit and would really concentrate on trying to help the baby's mother and the other staff through the weeks ahead. This is just what he in fact did, amazing the departmental head with his previously unseen maturity and concern for others. One or two other staff, however, took up the option of some short-term support with the counsellor.

FOLLOW-UP BY THE LINE MANAGER

Some of the follow up may be delegated to a human resources manager or whoever led the debriefing, but it is important that the line manager is also seen as personally committed to the well-being of the staff. He or she delegates that concern at their peril and needs to find ways of expressing it and checking out how people are from time to time. Then the debriefer or manager needs to ensure that there is follow up within a reasonable period, sooner rather than later. It is all too easy after such a debriefing to become caught up with other priorities and pressures, so that time slips by, forgetting that for the staff what happened may still be dominating their waking hours. The follow up, sorting out unfinished business, may be an important ingredient in staff being able to move on.

If staff are on prescribed medication as a result of the incident, there may be implications for their ability to work accurately and safely. Consultation with occupational health or their general practitioner, with the staff member's permission, may be appropriate before the person returns to full duties or, equally, before making changes to their job.

A FOLLOW-UP PERIOD OF ONE-TO-ONE COUNSELLING

As one of the further support options, counselling can be helpful, but must be understood as optional. This will be reinforced in the initial 'contracting' described in Chapter 4. On the other hand, the message should also be that it is not a sign of weakness to talk things over with a counsellor. The senior manager on site can set an example by letting the staff know that he or she is having a chat with the counsellor. Staff can be encouraged to have one session as a sort of personal insurance, on the basis that it should do no harm and may be useful, without being under pressure to continue beyond that if that is sufficient at the time, as it can be.

> One of Phil's sales team committed suicide in a side road on a day of visiting customers. Phil knew the round and went in search of him, when he failed to return or answer his mobile, and found his body. The first thing his boss said to him was how could they keep it out of the papers. He offered Phil nothing in the way of support.

Counsellors and managers, in emphasising the potential benefits of seeing a counsellor, need to avoid underestimating or undermining the support people at work can receive from each other. There is also a danger that some managers end up feeling unnecessarily deskilled by having a counsellor around. Consequently, an important role for the counsellor may be to support, help and affirm the manager in what they are doing, rather than take over the main support role from them.

> Isobel complained of feeling unwell and the branch manager, Peter, offered to take her home. When he got back to the office he mentioned to her sister Rachel, who also worked for the bank, that Isobel hadn't been feeling too well, and he had taken her home. They neither thought more of it, even though she had mentioned a slight pain in her chest. They were unaware that this can be a symptom of a heart attack. When Isobel's husband arrived home that evening he found that she had died during the day. Peter and especially Rachel were full of guilt that they had not followed up, and checked that she was all right during the day. She had always been so fit that they had never dreamt how serious her symptoms were.
> The company offered both Rachel and Peter some counselling support, which got them through the worst of it. It also helped them in

different ways, ensuring that Isobel's husband was supported as well as possible in turn. The counsellor also had one meeting with the two of them, which they found useful, as the shared guilt that they both felt had put a strain on their working relationship. Rachel originally felt that she could not go on working there, but the quality of the support she felt that she received from colleagues, as well as the counsellor, helped change her mind. Peter was especially pleased both because she was a valued and trustworthy member of staff and because there had been some resolution from such a painful episode.

After a traumatic incident, some one-to-one crisis support is often best offered in the first two or three weeks in the first instance. The number of sessions in many cases will be in single figures, and some staff will find one or two both useful and sufficient. If the company has an employee assistance programme, this would probably be in line with the number of sessions available to all staff with a counsellor. Employee assistance programme contracts tend to vary between four to 10 sessions as the norm.

After that, if more specialist support seems appropriate, a decision will need to be worked through with the human resources or senior line manager as to whether it is acceptable to the employer to allow time off and pay the cost of some further sessions. Good employers will not be rigid about this, but equally resources are limited and in practice such exceptions in my experience are not common. The options are, when extra support is appropriate, for the same counsellor to continue and be paid by the company or the counsellor might help the staff member link to a completely external counsellor or agency, in which case there might or might not be a fee to pay. Cruse Bereavement Care, for example, is a charity and offers one-to-one bereavement support from trained volunteers on a no-fee basis in many parts of Britain. They fund-raise energetically to cover the back-up needed to recruit, train and supervise their volunteers. Of course, such considerations may be different if the counsellor is a direct employee of the organisation and is paid a salary rather than a sessional fee.

While one-to-one support using counselling may not be needed nor wanted in those early days and weeks, something unresolved and troubling may keep nagging away and work its way through to the surface months or even a year later. So a member of staff may come to be glad that the offer is still open.

VISITS FROM SENIOR MANAGEMENT

Visits from senior management are often important after a traumatic death at work. Although they can be helpful, they can, however, also misfire and be counter-productive, depending on the way the senior management behave on the visit. The reputation of whoever visits and their preexisting relationship with staff can also be significant. If the chief executive, director or senior manager comes over as genuinely concerned, human, and not in a cloud of self-importance, the back-up felt by both the local manager and staff involved can be tremendous.

> Tony had given the impression of being very task centred and not much of a people person after his appointment as the new division director. The business was in a precarious state and he put in place a number of initiatives that involved moving some senior managers, a few out of the company. Then the general manager of one of the overseas branches was murdered, and Tony went straight out there, spending time with the management team, helping them pick up the pieces, and also with the manager's widower, making sure that they all got the support that they needed.
> One of the staff said later that they got to see Tony's humanity in a way that they might never have done, but for the tragedy. Indeed, Tony discovered some humanity in himself that he had not realised was there. He was deeply affected and said afterwards that it seemed obvious that he put other business issues on hold, which were so secondary in importance to doing what could be done to deal with such a great tragedy.

A trap for the top manager, distracted by many other pressing demands for his or her attention, can be to appear to be going through the motions, not really engaged at a human level with what has happened. Colin Parry[7] wrote of his disappointment with both John Major, the then Prime Minister, and John Smith, the late leader of the opposition, on their visit to Warrington after the IRA bomb that killed his young son Tim and Johnathan Ball in 1993.

> My disappointment with [them both] stemmed from the fact that neither man asked me anything other than the orthodox and polite question 'How are you?'. This question is rarely answered honestly. You know they don't expect a long and detailed reply and so you don't give one. This is the unspoken understanding between the questioner and the person being questioned and is part of the ritual in our polite society.

Colin described the different impact that his local MP, David Alton, and the Irish President, Mary Robinson, made through their ability to convey a genuine wish to hear his views and opinions. They also communicated a greater awareness of what had happened to the Parry family and how they had responded to the tragedy. The difference may be because of the greater interest of these two in the event, rather than concern for the people affected. John Major, for example, had taken the trouble immediately after Tim's death to write a sensitive and hand-written letter to the Parrys, model behaviour for a caring chief executive.

A chief executive going to a funeral or making a personal visit must take the trouble to be well briefed beforehand and to have thought about what to say and what to ask if the effort made is to be experienced as helpful. This applies to young people as well. Tim Parry's older brother, for example, was asked endlessly by visiting dignitaries what he wanted to do when he left school, as if they could not find a way of acknowledging his own loss.[8]

Sensitivity is also required of the top manager in relation to the line, human resources and other managers more directly involved. Top management involvement has to aim to reinforce, compliment and support, rather than outshine, the others. This has to be subtly interwoven with alertness to the overall adequacy of the company response to an extremely difficult situation.

Notes

1 National Centre for Post Traumatic Stress Disorder (1993) *Clinical Newsletter*, vol 3, no 1, Winter.
2 Parkinson, F. (1993) *Post Trauma Stress*, London: Sheldon.
3 BBC Radio 4 (1999) *File on 4*, 21 February.
4 BBC Radio 4 (1999), *ibid*.
5 Bergman, D. *Deaths at Work – Accidents Or Corporate Crime: The Failure Of Inquests and The Criminal Justice System*, London: The Workers' Educational Association.
6 Feltham, C. (ed) (1994) *The Gains of Listening: Perspectives on Counselling at Work*, Buckingham: Open University Press.
7 Parry, C. and Parry, W. (1994) *Tim: An Ordinary Boy*, London: Hodder and Stoughton.
8 Parry, C. and Parry, W. (1994), *ibid*.

Section 5

Case studies

Chapter 17

Case studies

- The death of a colleague and a friend
- The death of a partner
- The death of a father
- The death of a daughter

THE DEATH OF A COLLEAGUE AND A FRIEND

Daniel was an industrial relations manager in the motor industry. He had a deserved reputation for handling the pressure well of what at times were heated and tense negotiations about pay and conditions. But after the death of Bob, a friend who was also a colleague, Daniel became very low, finding it hard to concentrate and maintain his motivation to the point where his boss suggested it might be useful for him to see a counsellor. Daniel agreed and three strands emerged from the counselling, helping him regain his focus and energy.

Bob was a few years older than Daniel, and had been something of a father figure to him when he started in the company, guiding and encouraging him. Their working relationship grew into a friendship, in which they shared a passion for Aston Villa, and often a drink at the end of the day. The friendship matured into one much more of equals as Daniel grew in seniority and confidence, finding ways in which he could help Bob, especially in financial and taxation matters. But in talking about what Bob's friendship and his death had meant to him, Daniel found that the memories of how he had felt when his parents had died years before had also been stirred up. It was as if he was experiencing a double or even triple bereavement. This was particularly extreme, because he had not been able or been given the opportunity to grieve over their deaths. So he came to realise that he needed to focus on all three separately to allow him to move on through his grief.

Daniel's parents had separated 20 years previously, when he was 10. He and his brother lived with his mother in Bristol, losing contact with his father, who moved up north with a new job. After three years, when Daniel was 13, his mother collapsed in front of him, was rushed into hospital (after he alerted a neighbour) and died a week later.

Daniel's father reappeared in order to care for the children after his wife's death. After a predictably rocky start to the re-establishment of their relationship, father and son eventually became close, based on a sense of shared responsibility for keeping the family going, football and visits to the seaside. The mutual love between them, through ups and downs, gradually grew, until six years later, with a bitter irony, his father collapsed with a stroke in the same room in which his mother had been taken ill. Daniel began to lose his father again that day, even though he did not die for another two years. So he learned early that we can lose those to whom we are close. To make himself forget about the past and the pain associated with it, he removed everything that might remind him of it. To this day he has no photographs of his parents to show his own children and virtually nothing that belonged to either of them. He wishes that someone had encouraged him then to keep a few mementoes at least.

Bob's death reminded him, originally unconsciously, of the deaths of both his parents. It brought to the front of his mind how much he still missed his father. What came out of this painful awareness was the re-evaluation of his own relationship with his children in the present. He was allowing time with them to slip down his list of priorities. At the top of that list was work, work and yet more work. Re-evaluating all of this, he talked over his long hours with his boss, who had also become something of a workaholic, and gained his agreement to get home earlier at least two days a week in order to spend time with his family. He was also making opportunities to do things with his children in a way that he had previously failed to do.

Bereavement counselling is not desirable for everyone who is bereaved, but in Daniel's case it helped to disentangle the threads of three losses, spread over 20 years. Individually they were manageable, but together added up to a bewildering mountain of grief, which initially felt overwhelming.

Daniel's line manager was astute enough to see that counselling might help and Daniel accepted the offer, because he realised that he was feeling so low: his motivation had dived. It also helped that he had participated in an introduction to counselling skills residential workshop for all the senior members of the human resources department a few years before. The workshop had dispelled some of his fears and suspicions about counselling, and made it easier to contemplate using the process without feeling that he was being weak.

THE DEATH OF A PARTNER

Sarah's career as research chemist was going well with her recent promotion to a senior managerial role in the laboratory, even while she was still just the right side of 40. At home she was, on the whole, happy, although her relationship with Barrie was going through a mildly difficult patch.

They both worked long hours and his shifts meant their time together was minimal and often fraught. But they stuck to their commitment of keeping Sundays clear, when he wasn't working. And then suddenly the rug was pulled from under their feet, when he was diagnosed from motor neurone disease.

As Barrie progressively became more incapacitated, previous tensions between them evaporated: they seemed so trivial in the face of the challenges they were now facing. Her parents lived nearby and helped care for him while she was at work. A district nurse and Macmillan nurse added to the support that they needed. Barrie also paid a weekly visit to the day unit of the local hospice, and greatly appreciated the physical and emotional support he received there, not least the special bath and Jacuzzi.

For Sarah, the three years until Barrie's death were a constant juggling of being open and reticent both at work and home, expressing and denying how she felt. The thought that they had had of children was terminated with his diagnosis, which upset them both in addition to the myriad issues they had to face about the present and future. Barrie had always had an enquiring mind and soon knew virtually as much as the doctors and nurses about his illness and prognosis so they were realistic about the likely journey that they were taking together.

Barrie's parents lived further away and they saw less of them. They were older and not much help in terms of looking after him. Both sets of parents, however, were unable or unwilling to countenance anything but unrealistic optimism about his future. Most of her colleagues, with whom she worked closely, except Diana, also played the same tune.

Diana was a relief. When she asked Sarah how she was feeling, there was something about how she asked her and the kind of person she was that enabled Sarah to answer straightforwardly and honestly. She did not feel she had to reassure or protect Diana, who did not over-react when Sarah was feeling low. Diana never seemed to make the situation worse, and often helped it feel slightly better even on the darkest of days. The most helpful conversations were often quite short, and on many days enabled Sarah to do some useful work after arriving feeling completely incapable with weariness or misery.

Work was a very mixed blessing. Before motor neurone disease entered their lives, Sarah had thought of herself as pretty 'emotionally literate'. In some meetings, however, she found herself in a 'Catch 22'. If other people were talking for most of the time, her mind might wander back to Barrie and she might become tearful, apparently unpredictably to others. Her well-founded fear was that some of her colleagues might start to characterise her as not being able to cope and a little unstable, quite understandably, of course, in view of what she was going through, but nevertheless a little unstable.

Sarah struggled with the question about whether or not to give up her job. A bit of her was drawn to give it up and give all her time to caring for Barrie, as his mother strongly intimated that she should. On the other hand, they needed the money and she in some ways felt that she needed her work psychologically as well as financially. Her line manager left her to it. He was embarrassed about the whole thing and took the line that his door was always open if she wanted to talk about anything with him. The human resources manager was also emotionally absent. Sarah wasn't a union member, so she survived with Diana as her unofficial shop steward. At times, she worried about leaning too heavily on her but was mostly just glad she was there. What reassured Sarah most of all was the full life Diana continued to pursue socially and with other interests outside work.

Sarah knew that she and Barrie were in great turmoil. She had no belief in any life after death, although he thought and certainly hoped that in some way they would meet again, not that that made their imminent parting easier. His illness made communication, as well as virtually everything else for him, increasingly difficult.

In the end, Sarah did take three months leave, at first annual. When she approached her line manager about staying away at the end of the first week, he came through very supportively and reassured her that she must put Barrie first and that the work would wait. He would sort out with human resources some leave whereby her pay would not be affected one way or another for a month or two. Barrie died towards the beginning of the third month.

Sarah felt very grateful at the way her manager behaved at this stage: it wasn't primarily the money, although that helped considerably alleviate anxiety, but his attitude that she valued. When Sarah started to come back to work, he continued to come in out of the cold and started to talk with her more openly and even at times on his own initiative. It was as if his embarrassment had gone with Barrie's death. She was touched and surprised that he and Diana came to the funeral, slipping off after the service. Meanwhile, Diana continued to be a pillar of strength during the early weeks, but fortunately other colleagues also seemed less tongue-tied with her than before. Work became an anchor in her journey of mourning.

THE DEATH OF A FATHER

The four farm cottages made an excellent base for a holiday in the country-side, not far from the sea. You needed to book well in advance if you wanted to rent one during the summer. Easter and Whitsun bookings were picking up, although they tended to be empty for most of the year. George, still active in his late seventies, ran the holiday cottages as a part-time retire-ment job. It brought in some extra income to the farm, which was under increasing economic pressures. Their milk now fetched a third of the price of three years ago.

George had been born in the farmhouse in which he still lived with his son, Robert. His wife had died five years previously, six months before their golden wedding. When George started working on the farm, helping his father, there were 10 men. Now Robert did it all on his own with occasional help from one nomadic farm worker during harvest time. Working with a tractor and earmuffs was both faster and also more isolated than with the long-gone team of horses.

Then one day, George had a heart attack and died.

Robert then had to contend with isolation in his bereavement that was different to that experienced by previous generations of his family. The farm, his workplace, seemed very empty. There was no human company on the farm, now that he did not have his father to argue with or consult, depending on the mood of the moment. He felt glad that he was not just an arable farmer, and found some comfort in the companionship of their animals, especially his two dogs. The vicar, based in a village five miles away, did his best but Robert hardly knew him. Like many of his generation, he felt alienated from the church, though his parents had been involved: his mother had run the choir and been active in the Mother's Union. He thought about going again after the funeral, but decided against it. He was busy and doubted if he believed half of what was said in the services.

In some ways, George's death was a relief. He was glad that both his parents had had their '3 score years and 10' and been spared debilitating final illnesses. They had both died at home, as they had wanted. Furthermore, in their case, two had seemed to make less congenial company than three. After his mother's death, Robert found his father got on his nerves more than he used to. On the other hand, the isolation really got to him, and he was surprised by his misery, which was a lot more than when his mother died. His father's death not only severed their link but also his last link with her too. So he ended up grieving for them both. And it was hard doing it all on his own. He and his father never cried in front of each other when his mother died, but they talked about her a lot. There was no one to talk to now.

Robert began to feel he understood why so many farmers seemed to end up killing themselves. What was the point of going on living? He had never felt like that before, and had been baffled when, two years before, a neighbour took his car into the hills one day and fitted a hose to the exhaust. At the time he had thought that farmers were a tough lot and was fond of the saying: 'when the going gets tough, the tough get going'. So Robert did not end it all. He felt that he had a reason to go on living, although he was not sure that he could put it into words.

Slowly he worked through the bereavement process in his own way, cursing and grumbling as he got out of bed in the morning and went about keeping the farm going, rattling around in a farmhouse designed for a family. But it was the loneliness of bereavement that impacted on him with most force. It did not help that it mirrored and reinforced the increasing isolation of his workplace. The pub helped and his place in the local darts team: he was smart and disciplined enough not to drink more than he used to, not that he had ever enjoyed alcohol that much. So that temptation wasn't strong. But at work, Robert had to take what support he could: largely from his own company, the familiar countryside, the farm animals and his sheepdogs, which were great listeners and totally trustworthy with his innermost thoughts and feelings that he would not share with anyone else.

THE DEATH OF A DAUGHTER

It was a dense foggy evening in early December, when Ian's youngest child Nicola had her accident. She was only 24 when it happened. She and her partner had recently moved into a new home, a cottage in the country 15 miles from where she worked. Visibility that night was down to a few yards, and the lane down which they lived had no lighting or road markings. Apparently she missed her way and drove off the road into a tree. A neighbour who saw the wreck shortly afterwards, called the emergency services but Nicola was dead by the time that the ambulance arrived.

Ian and his wife Brenda were shaken to their roots, but somehow got through the few weeks afterwards. They had been helped by the support they were able to give and, even more, receive from Nicola's partner and some of her close friends, who they had known for years. These young people spoke and made music at the funeral, and made them realise how special a human being they also thought their daughter was. Some of them took to dropping in frequently on Ian and Brenda for endless cups of this and that round their kitchen table, when they would reminisce about Nicola. It was as if all their lives had come to a full stop. The younger generation seemed a lot less inhibited than they were, but they all had a sense of shared grief and support by maintaining contact.

At work, Ian felt gutted, but relieved how well he was handling it, at least at first, but he was worried about Brenda. She and Nicola had had an almost telepathic relationship, and had always stayed very close. She seemed to miss out on her adolescent rebellion, which was mostly concentrated in a couple of years of struggle with her father, but that had soon abated after she left home to go to college. Since then, Nicola's friendship with both parents had become relaxed as well as strong.

Ian encouraged Brenda to talk to their general practitioner, who had put her on anti-depressants and pointed her towards a counsellor. She had some good women friends, not least at the council offices where she worked as a section leader in the housing department. Brenda's line manager encouraged her to take her time in coming back to work. 'I know that you are only human, so you are bound to be miles away from time to time, even if you are at your desk. So don't worry, and don't give yourself a hard time. None of us will.' She still felt pretty battered, but did not expect anything else, given what had happened.

Six months later, Brenda felt that she was coming up for air, but things suddenly seemed not so good for Ian. In the aftermath of the tragedy, he had seemed so strong, holding the family together, even though, as it always had, his work took him away from home quite a bit. His senior position in an advertising agency, where he had worked for 20 years, involved quite a few clients based outside the UK. After he got back to work a couple of weeks after Nicola's death, he had assured his boss that, as far as he was concerned, to work normally would be the most helpful policy. His colleagues, all men with most of whom he had worked for years, were concerned for him. But they did not really know what to say and so they got on with their work. Neither he nor they initiated conversations about his daughter's death.

His boss became increasingly worried about him. The quality of his work slowly deteriorated and his interpersonal skills became unpredictable. He was more irritable than he used to be. Some of his colleagues shared their concerns about him with their line manager. He had become a byword in the company for his ability. In the past few months, however, he had lost some of his edge and it seemed to be getting worse. Was he just running out of steam? How much was it tied up, if at all, with his daughter's death. Surely he should be starting to get over it by now?

That was the gist of what Ian's boss shared with the human resources director, who suggested that as he had had a few months to work through his bereavement, it might be useful to offer him some counselling. Surprisingly Ian accepted the suggestion on the basis that it would probably be a waste of time but it couldn't do any harm, and he knew that he felt that he was sinking.

What emerged from the counselling was that he had not really talked to anybody, except Brenda, about what he was going through, certainly not his male friends, who conspired to try and cheer him up at all costs, and that was backfiring. If he refused to be cheered, he felt that they became impatient with him and he with them. Because he felt that Brenda's grief was greater than his, he minimised his own grief with her (and to an extent with himself), rather than risk upsetting her more than she was already. He talked a lot with the counsellor about his family and Nicola's life and her death. What also came to the surface was how much, like so many others, he had missed out in terms of time with her and his other children and his home. When he was based at home, the working hours had meant he had only seen the children awake at weekends until they were teenagers. Even quite a lot of weekends were lost to the many trips abroad.

Work had had its own impetus and bowled him along, and he had never really stopped to think about his priorities. Her death was forcing to the surface of his mind a re-evaluation of the time and the energy he spent at home and at work. Bereavement made Ian rethink his workaholic life and values. It led to a decision nine months later to take an early retirement option, to which he was entitled. It meant some careful calculations and equally careful discussion with Brenda, because there were significant financial consequences in retiring early. He told the human resources director when sorting out the details of his departure: 'I guess we cannot have a tragedy like this happen and just steam on as if nothing had happened. It's got to me in ways I just didn't expect'. Before his daughter's death, neither Ian, Brenda nor his colleagues would ever have imagined such a decision from 'the old Ian'. A year later he and Brenda had pulled in their financial horns a bit but were very glad that they had made that decision.

Section 6

Appendices

Appendix 1

Checklists

Please feel free to copy any of the following checklists:

- A checklist for the bereaved person
- A checklist for helping bereaved children
- A checklist for the organisation: support over the funeral
- A checklist for the bereaved person: returning to work
- A checklist for colleagues: when a bereaved person returns to work
- A checklist for friends, relatives and neighbours: how to support people during bereavement

In Chapter 9, there are also two notes from the Samaritans:

- How can I spot someone at risk of suicide?
- Signs of suicide risk: what can I do?

A CHECKLIST FOR THE BEREAVED PERSON

If someone close to you has died, it may be helpful to know how others have coped in similar situations, even though your experience is unique. These notes draw together some points that tie into the experience of other people.

Your feelings

The emotional pain of bereavement is very strong and unavoidable: its depth will be a reflection of how deeply you loved or cared for the person who has died. If death came after an illness that you (and perhaps the person) knew was terminal, you may already have started the process of mourning (or healing the pain of loss). But, however much you imagine you are prepared for someone's death, the actual experience often makes you feel that you have not really anticipated it at all. If the person died suddenly and unexpectedly, there may be a more prolonged period of shock (when it may be hard to take in what has happened) before the grieving begins.

Normal feelings

It is usual to experience, often very strongly, a mixture of feelings, coming one after the other repeatedly, although not necessarily in this order:

- shock and numbness
- longing
- sadness or depression
- disappointment
- anger and resentment
- relief
- loneliness
- fear
- helplessness
- freedom and emancipation
- guilt, shame or regret
- hope and despair
- happy memories
- resignation or acceptance.

Your dreams

A sense of unreality can pervade your waking life but also your sleep, which may be disturbed. Even if you do not normally remember your dreams, you may now recall vivid dreams, perhaps bad ones. They may make a lot of sense, or not much at all. These dreams are a method by which the unconscious mind works over the feelings mentioned in the previous section, sorting them out while the conscious part of the mind is at rest.

Your body's response

Your body responds to bereavement as well as your mind. You may frequently experience such physical sensations as:

- sleeplessness
- breathing difficulties
- headaches, dry mouth, hollowness in the stomach and other discomfort
- tiredness and lack of energy
- dizziness
- diarrhoea and nausea
- difficulty in concentrating and remembering things
- social withdrawal and/or periods of being overactive.

If you are concerned about any of these symptoms, it may be helpful to consult your doctor, but make sure that you mention your bereavement.

The healing process

Your body, mind and 'heart' need to be healed from the shock and pain of your loss. This happens naturally, if you let it and allow yourself time. The quality of support you receive from family and friends is important: sometimes the healing process needs others present as you share or work through your feelings, although sometimes you may want to be alone.

Sharing your feelings with another person who is not too closely involved can also at times, for some people, be very helpful, since you will feel less obliged to protect them from how you are really feeling. This is why bereavement counselling can be useful – often after some time has passed.

If your pain heals, it does not mean that you did not care enough in the first place. If you loved the person deeply or valued them as a colleague, there will always be a gap in your heart. Healing means that you start to be able to feel normal again, and to feel whole, without the person being with you. This may mean that you have begun to take something of their qualities and personality into yourself.

Emotional healing happens through:

- allowing yourself to 'feel the feelings', and perhaps to share how you really feel with a trusted person. You may need to think and talk about what you particularly treasure about the person who has died, the relationship you had and your memories of times together, both good and bad.
- being prepared to do this thinking and talking again and again. It may seem like repetition, but it is never quite the same and this kind of healing takes time and going over the same ground.
- letting your body 'feel the feelings' as well as your mind. You can do this through talking with feeling or passion, through laughing, crying, raging, shaking and yawning. Don't stop your body from doing those things. Let your body express itself, when and where it feels safe to do so, on your own and also with people you trust.
- while avoiding bottling feelings up, do not feel you have to go into detail about how you are feeling just because someone asks you. Reticence is also fine and you can work out a reply that is true for you but not too long, such as 'Thanks for asking. It's pretty tough at times, but I am getting there'.

Time-scales

How long will it take? Talk about time-scales for 'recovery' is best avoided because each situation is unique and so generalisations are difficult. But two points can be emphasised:

- Mourning someone close to you is not a short-term process. The overwhelming aspects of acute grief may loosen their grip intermittently after a few days, but the full process can take months, even years. A sign of moving forward is the re-occurrence of periods when you feel more normal, even like you used to feel. When painful feelings return, however, they can often be as intense as ever.

■ If after a few months you still feel constantly overwhelmed by extreme grief, it may help to consult someone, if you have not already done so: for example, a counsellor, your local branch of Cruse, the Gay Bereavement Project, your family doctor, the Samaritans or someone at the local church, mosque, synagogue or temple.

Don't be surprised, however, if at times you still feel devastated long after the person has died. Poignant memories and reminders – visits to old haunts, photographs, letters, birthdays, Christmas and other anniversaries – can all trigger a sense of acute grief. Some people get worried if they still feel low just a couple of weeks after a bereavement, but the process of mourning doesn't come to an end when compassionate leave is over and you return to work.

Others who are grieving, especially children

If there are other people also deeply affected by the loss, it may help them if you find out how they are feeling. There is a measure of healing simply in good listening, with discretion and free from the fear of gossip. This is especially important for children: they grieve too and will need to talk and sometimes to express their feelings, perhaps through games and drawings, especially when they are young. If you are a parent, do not hide all your grief from your children. If, because you are shielding them from it, they are not aware of it, they may feel that you don't care, and then can feel unnecessarily isolated in their own loss.

Safety

Because bereavement affects levels of stress and tiredness, you will need to watch yourself and others with respect to safety at home and work. In particular, drive carefully. Warn children to be careful, and be less inclined than usual to blame them if they do have an accident. They need extra support too, like you do, even if it's a different kind.

Be careful if you are increasing your consumption of alcohol or nicotine. Apart from the safety and health implications, they will not actively assist the healing process, and can even impede it. They may numb painful feelings for a short time, but not for long.

Practicalities

Allow yourself more time than usual to do things at home and work. Be more prepared than usual to accept offers of help, including matters relating to the bereavement. These may include:

- registering the death
- letting people know
- decisions, such as:

  - where the body should be
  - cremation or burial
  - where the ashes should go
  - other funeral arrangements

- letters and callers
- pension, insurance and other financial matters
- personal possessions.

But give yourself time over decisions. It is often best to defer major decisions about the future – if that is possible. This is no time to hurry unless it is really essential.

Work

Consider your colleagues as potential resources for emotional and practical help. If they offer help, either accept it or at least do not automatically refuse; take their telephone number and be prepared to call them, if you feel the offer was genuine. If colleagues can help, they act as a bridge between you and the workplace. It may be important to have such a bridge in place after a bereavement.

If you have not already done so, arrange to meet your supervisor before you return to work or as soon as possible on returning, so that you can talk things over.

Take as much time off work as you feel you need and are permitted. If your compassionate leave allowance seems inadequate, talk it over with your line manager and/or someone in personnel or welfare, or your trades union representative. If, after that, you still feel that you need more time, discuss it with your GP who may decide to 'sign you off' for a while.

Pace your return to work in consultation with your supervisor. Here are two possibilities worth considering:

- It may be possible to return initially on a part-time basis, say for the first week or two.
- Recognise that your concentration and capacity for creative thought will be below par at first. Some relatively easy, undemanding work may be a good way of easing you back in.

If you have someone at work that you can trust, continue well after the bereavement to talk to this person (or people) about how it is going for you.

Remember that some painful feelings may return, long after the bereavement, as powerful and as devastating as ever. This does not mean that you are failing to make progress. At times grieving can feel a bit like going round in circles; but accepting, and going with it, is the way through. What it probably suggests is that you need to complete one more bit of grieving, and that you are ready to do so.

A CHECKLIST FOR HELPING BEREAVED CHILDREN

- Listen and notice carefully with your eyes as well as ears.
- Be perhaps even more sensitive about timing than with adults.
- Let them be distracted, get on with their life the way they want to.
- Offer to talk and provide full and clear information.
- Be prepared not to push it or yourself.
- Be alert to and willing to address their fears and anxieties.
- Acknowledge and respect the child's feelings.
- Reassure them that they will be cared for.
- Be alert to the fear that a remaining parent (or they) will die.
- Maintain consistency of care, not inappropriate lax discipline.
- Be prepared to reassure them that they are not to blame, and that the person did not want to leave them.
- Discuss the death and the person sensitively, naturally and openly so that the child can do the same, when they want to.
- Give the child time and the opportunity to remember the dead person before being encouraged to sever bonds a little in order to get on with their life.
- Be honest, not least about your own beliefs, uncertainties or lack of belief in an after-life and that they will not return in this life.
- Do not be afraid to show some of your own feelings, including tears, in front of the child: it may make them feel less disturbed about how they feel.
- Do not minimise their sadness over the death of a pet, or other losses.
- Be careful about praising them for being brave or pressurising them to be brave and not to express how they really feel.
- Help them express how they feel in different ways about the person and/or their death, for example through drawings, sculpting in clay, poetry, other writing and different forms of play.
- Let them write letters to the deceased in the present tense, if they wish.
- Help them, if they want, to produce a scrapbook of memories, using drawings, pictures, press cuttings, photos and their own and perhaps others' writings.
- Create and notice opportunities to remember and celebrate the person who has died, such as birthdays and other anniversaries, so that their memory is not buried and forgotten.
- Be prepared for the possibility that they might be helped by some further, perhaps external support, especially but not exclusively within the first two years.

A CHECKLIST FOR THE ORGANISATION: SUPPORT OVER THE FUNERAL

Offer, via the line manager, a human resources person or other suitable company representative, contact before the funeral, if possible with a visit to establish any or all of the following:

- Does the next-of-kin need support for planning what to do immediately?
- Do they need money urgently to help pay for expenses?
- What are the wishes of the deceased or immediate family?
- Would they like a book from the company for attendees at the funeral to sign? If so, keep the company aspect low key in the book.
- Any other ways in which the company could help?

Consider the following issues as well:

- Who at work needs to be informed (and how) and who might attend the funeral?
- Time off to be arranged sensitively.
- Any transport implications?
- Anyone whom the next-of-kin particularly want (or do not want) to attend?
- A personally signed letter from the most senior person appropriate to the next-of-kin, expressing appreciation of the deceased as well as condolences.
- A donation to the specified charity or flowers to be sent: if flowers, do not make them ostentatious so that they do not overshadow those from close family or friends.

A CHECKLIST FOR THE BEREAVED PERSON: RETURNING TO WORK

Do

- Let yourself experience the pain of grief.
- Share how you feel with those (including colleagues) with whom you feel safe, choosing time and place.
- Allow yourself more rest than usual: bereavement can be very tiring.
- Avoid heavy drinking (or illegal drugs) to dull the pain.
- Be cautious about major decisions in the early months.
- Expect the need to talk about your loss to continue for longer than you might expect.
- Break yourself in gently and gradually after a discussion with your manager.
- Be prepared to ask for permission in the early days especially to go for a walk from your work station if you feel overcome and need breathing space for a few minutes.

- Try and be open about the kind of support that you want (and don't want).

Don't

- Try to avoid the pain.
- Be ashamed of your feelings – or tears.
- Fight the need to talk about it over and over again.
- Return to work until you feel you are ready.
- Take on new tasks or responsibilities too quickly.
- Be surprised if your concentration is affected.
- Be surprised if you have vivid and grief dreams.
- Be ashamed of your grief: it's a consequence of your friendship and love.

A CHECKLIST FOR COLLEAGUES: WHEN A BEREAVED PERSON RETURNS TO WORK

Do

- Respect their reticence and their openness.
- Acknowledge the loss. Care more about the person than your own embarrassment.
- Encourage the person to talk, if they want to.
- Enable people to cry without loss of safety or self-respect.
- Reassure them that very powerful, vivid and unfamiliar feelings and dreams are a normal part of grieving.
- Check whether close colleagues know of the bereavement.
- Check whether the bereaved wants others to be informed (who and how?).
- Acknowledge important anniversaries suitably and sensitively (deaths as well as births, weddings, etc.).
- Discourage people from taking major decisions (job change, house move, etc.) early in the bereavement.

Don't

- Pressurise them to get on with work if it is not essential.
- Minimise the impact of the loss.
- Reassure, when what's needed is permission to share grief.
- Limit the time in which support is given.
- Expect bereaved colleagues to be 'back to normal' quickly.
- Let your embarrassment stop you offering support.

A CHECKLIST FOR FRIENDS, RELATIVES AND NEIGHBOURS: HOW TO SUPPORT PEOPLE DURING BEREAVEMENT

- Encourage (but do not bully or push) them to talk about the person who has died and how they died.
- Share your own memories of the person who has died.
- Enable them to cry without loss of safety or self-respect.
- Encourage them to talk about the support (or lack of it) – good and bad – that they are receiving.
- Consider making telephone calls to check out how they are, perhaps in the not-too-early morning and give them permission to telephone you whenever they feel the need, including during the night.
- Offer, if needed, practical help or teaching tasks, such as cooking or car maintenance, which their spouse previously undertook.
- Encourage them to revisit old haunts when they are ready, asking how it was and/or accompanying them.
- Support (but don't rush) them to take up new interests, make new friends, etc. – when the time is right.
- Warn them that it may not be wise to take major decisions, e.g. house moves, remarriage, job changes, etc., during the early few months of bereavement.
- Be around after the funeral and immediate period of mourning, when other family and friends tend to disappear.
- Be aware of danger signals, e.g. prolonged anorexia, heavy drinking, withdrawal, etc., which indicate the need for more expert help.
- Reassure them that vivid dreams, talking to the deceased, forgetting not to lay his or her place at the table, etc., are all quite normal – there can be an undue fear of insanity at this time.
- Remember anniversaries (e.g. death, birthday, wedding) and find a sensitive way of acknowledging them.
- Provide companionship and friendship, where it may be needed, at work and/or outside.

Appendix 2

The core conditions of helping

'The Core Conditions of Helping' have been identified as an excellent, necessary and sufficient basis for good relationships. They are important in teams as well as one-to-one relationships. They can be easily remembered by an accessible acronym *GUM*: G for Genuineness (and honesty), U for Understanding (and empathy, communicating understanding) and M for Mutual Respect (and acceptance). They are associated originally with the work of Carl Rogers and the development of person-centred counselling, but have a much wider application than that.[1] They are crucial in supporting those who are bereaved or terminally ill in whatever role. They are on one level so simple and yet so often they are significantly absent in working relationships.

- *Genuineness* or congruence is the capacity to be straight, to be yourself and not hide behind a mask of some kind, such as your role, or to play devious games. By being genuine, permission is given implicitly to the other person that they can also be real and themselves in that relationship. The sense that someone is pretending to care in the face of bereavement, but actually does not care at all, is very alienating. The more genuine you are, the more likely you are to be yourself whether at home or in different work settings, rather than switching your genuineness on and off, depending on who you are with. The possible cost of being genuine is that, by not putting up the barricades of self-protecting, false professionalism, you too will be affected and perhaps upset as well in the face of other people's distress. Some find it hard to be genuine with certain people because of a lack of self-confidence. Such confidence can be built in a variety of ways, depending on your particular needs: through accepting yourself, as well as other people; through assertiveness; through strengthening support; and through high-quality feedback. An anxiety that prevents some being genuine is the fear that their authority may be undermined by a lack of 'distance' between them and their staff; but over-familiarity and being genuine are not the same. While, at times, leadership may require detachment and objectivity in considering people and problems, they need to be combined with humanity. Honesty has been identified as the key attribute wanted by staff of their managers and also came top of the list of qualities often thought to be lacking. People want to trust their managers and to feel that they are genuine, particularly at times of personal difficulty or vulnerability. Sometimes that may mean the manager has to admit that they do not know what to say or do for the best.

■ *Empathy* is the ability to communicate *understanding* and to see a situation from another person's point of view. The key skills for understanding are listening and reflecting. The worst stereotype of leadership is one in which the leader dominates by talking, if not shouting, while the led listen: for such a leader to listen with respect to subordinates would be a sign of weakness, because the leader should also have a monopoly of wisdom. Such a model gives leadership a bad name. Listening leaders understand and respect their people and appreciate that each of them has a unique perspective on their own job, which maybe no one else has. Their suggestions on how to do the job better and also on broader issues for the company are worth taking seriously, even if there may be reasons for not acting on all their recommendations. Such a leader does not need to be indecisive. In the context of serious illness or bereavement, managers and colleagues who have developed their empathy skills are likely to be more effective in support than those who have not.

■ *Effective listening* is vital from a manager or supervisor, who is with a staff member coming to terms with their own or someone else's death. It is achieved through the eyes and the whole body, not just the ears, because it involves non-verbal communication. If you are not looking at the person while you listen, you risk giving the impression that you are not really listening whole-heartedly with interest and respect. You also risk missing some important non-verbal clues, which may add to your understanding, especially about how the person feels. Reflecting is an essential component of listening through reflecting back what the person is essentially saying and also often acknowledging how they are feeling. Too often, people listen without looking and restrict their verbal inputs to questioning, without reflecting: such listening lacks competence, empathy and encouragement.

■ *Mutual respect* or acceptance involves an acceptance of and respect for people as human beings, without any sense of intrinsic superiority over them on the basis of status, qualifications, race, tribe, age, gender, sexual orientation, state of health or for any other reason. Mutual respect also implies a commitment to staff as people. If I feel that the organisation, through my manager, is committed to my health, welfare and success, I am more likely to reciprocate through my commitment to the health, welfare and success of the company through the simple principle of 'Do as you would be done by'.

Mutual respect also reminds us of the interdependence of everyone in the organisation for its success, whatever job you happen to occupy at the moment. Such respect for the person needs to underpin and be stronger than respect for their effectiveness and output, not least when they are adversely affected by illness or bereavement, albeit mostly in the short term. On the other hand, respect does not mean colluding or agreeing with or failing to challenge unacceptable behaviour or differing views to your own, nor shirking from disciplinary action, if and when required. In the latter instance, it does mean distinguishing in your own mind and behaviour between the person you are disciplining who is as worthy of respect as you are, and their behaviour or performance, which is a cause of concern. That sense of respect may be the crucial ingredient that makes it possible for the person to respond undefensively to the points you are making and retain enough motivation and energy to act on it constructively. Disciplinary action needs, of course, to be even more a last resort in times of bereavement than it would in normal times.

The core conditions of helping underpin and complement rather than contradict the need for action and doing. How we lead is as important as what we do. Max De Pree, a successful chairperson of an American company, put it differently: 'Leaders owe the organisation a new reference point for what caring, purposeful, committed people can be in the institutional setting. Notice I did not say what people can do – what people can do is merely a consequence of what we can be. Corporations, like the people who compose them, are always in a state of becoming'.[2] The core conditions provide an essential, sound foundation on which to build effective leadership, motivation and teamwork in organisations that are human in the best sense of the word.

Notes

1   Mearns, D. and Thorne, B. (1999) *Person-centred Counselling in Action* (2nd edn), London: Sage Publications.
2   De Pree, M. (1989) *Leadership is an Art*, New York, NY: Doubleday.

Further reading

Death and bereavement has been written about extensively from many angles. The following is a selection:

ANTHOLOGIES

Albery, N., Nicholas, E., Elliot, G. and Elliot, J. (eds) (1997) *The New Natural Death Handbook*, London: Rider.
Saunders, C. (1983) *Beyond All Pain: A Companion for the Suffering and Bereaved*, London: SPCK.
Whitaker, A. (ed) (1984) *All in the End is Harvest: An Anthology for Those Who Grieve*, London: DLT/Cruse.

DEATH AND BEREAVEMENT – GENERAL

Ainsworth-Smith, I. and Speck, P. (1982) *Letting Go: Caring for the Dying and Bereaved*, London: SPCK.
Charles-Edwards, A. (1983) *The Nursing Care of the Dying Patient*, Beaconsfield: Beaconsfield Publishers.
De Hennezel, M. (1997) *Intimate Death: How the Dying Teach us to Live*, London: Little, Brown and Company.
Dickenson, D. and Johnson, M. (eds) (1993) *Death, Dying & Bereavement*. London: Sage Publications with the Open University.
Kubler-Ross, E. (1973) *On Death and Dying*, London: Tavistock.
Maxwell, C. (1989) 'Bereavement counselling', *Journal of Workplace Learning*, vol 5, no 2.
Murray Parkes, C. (1986) *Bereavement: Studies of Grief in Adult Life*, Harmondsworth: Pelican.
Nutall, N. (1991) *The Early Days of Grieving*, Beaconsfield: Beaconsfield Publishers.
Poss, S. (1981) *Towards Death with Dignity*, London: George Allen & Unwin.
Raphael, B. (1982) *The Anatomy of Bereavement*, London: Hutchinson.
Stedeford, A. (1984) *Facing Death: Patients, Families and Professionals*, London: Heinemann Medical.
Tatelbaum, J. (1981) *The Courage to Grieve*, London: Heinemann.
Thompson, N. (ed) (2002) *Loss and Grief: A Guide for Human Services Practitioners*, Basingstoke and New York, NY: Palgrave. [This book covers other loss situations in addition to death and dying, such as poverty, divorce, etc.]
Worden, W. (1983) *Grief Counselling and Grief Therapy*, London: Tavistock.

BEREAVEMENT, RELATIONSHIPS AND THE FAMILY

Pincus, L. (1976) *Death and the Family: The Importance of Mourning*, London: Faber.

Shuchter, S.R. (1986) *Dimensions of Grief: Adjusting to the Death of a Spouse*, London: Jossey-Bass.

Staudacher, C. (1991) *Men & Grief*, Oakland, CA: New Harbinger Publications.

BEREAVEMENT AND CHILDREN

Black, D. et al (1993) *Father Kills Mother: Post-Traumatic Stress Disorder in the Children*, London: Cruse Bereavement Care.

Bowlby, J. (1980) *Attachment and Loss: Loss, Sadness and Depression*, New York, NY: Basic Books.

Dominica, Sister Frances (1997) *Just My Reflection: Helping Parents To Do Things Their Way When Their Child Dies*, London: DLT.

Jewett, C. (1982) *Helping Children Cope with Separation and Loss: Childcare Policy and Practice*, London: B.T. Batsford.

Merrington, B. (1996) *Suffering Love: Coping with the Death of a Child*, Leamington Spa: Advantage.

Worden, W. (1996) *Children and Grief*, New York and London: Guildford Press.

PERSONAL ACCOUNTS OF BEREAVEMENT AND DYING

Ashenburg, K. (2003) *The Mourner's Dance*, New York, NY: North Point Press.

Blacker, T. (1998) 'The spirituality of sad old hippies', *The Independent*, 15 December.

De Beauvoir, S. (1995) *A Very Easy Death*, London: Andre Deutsch and Weidenfeld and Nicholson.

Dodson, J. (1997) *Final Rounds: Father, Son, the Golf Journey of a Lifetime*, London: Arrow Books.

Lewis, C.S. (1961) *A Grief Observed*, London: Faber & Faber.

Parry, C. and Parry, W. (1994) *Tim: An Ordinary Boy*, London: Hodder and Stoughton.

Payne, S. (2004) *A Mother's Story*, London: Hodder & Stoughton.

BEREAVEMENT, DEATH, CULTURE AND RELIGION

Baynes, A. (1992) 'What happens when we die?', in *The Buddhism of Nichiren Daishonin*.

Clark, D. (1993) *The Sociology of Death: Theory, Culture and Practice*, Oxford: Blackwells.

Collins, D., Tank, M. and Basith, A. (1992) *Concise Guide to Customs of Minority Ethnic Religions*, Portsmouth: Portsmouth Diocesan Council for Social Responsibility.

Cruse, *Best of Bereavement Care*, No 6, Cultural and Religious Aspects, London: Cruse.

Ikeda, D. (2003) *Unlocking the Mysteries of Birth and Death* (2nd edn), Santa Monica, CA: Middleway Press.

Gersie, A. (1991) *Storymaking in Bereavement: Dragons Fight in the Meadow*, London: Jessica Kingsley Publishers.

Gorer, G. (1965) *Death, Grief and Mourning*, London: Crescent.

Jacobs, L. (1973) *What does Judaism Say About?*, Jerusalem: Keter.

Knight, M. (1961) *Humanist Anthology from Confucius to Bertrand Russell*, London: Barrie & Rockliff for The Rationalist Press.

Laungani, M. (1997) *Death and Bereavement Across Cultures*, London: Routledge.

Murray Parkes, C., Laungani, P. and Young, B. (eds) (1996) *Death and Bereavement Across Cultures*, London: Routledge.

O'Donoghue, J. (1997) *Anam Cara: Spiritual Wisdom in the Celtic World*, London: Bantam Books.

Robinson, J.A.T. (1979) *Truth is Two-Eyed*, London: SCM Press.

Smart, N. (1968) 'Death in the Judaeo-Christian Tradition', in A. Toynbee et al (eds) *Man's Concern with Death*, London: Hodder & Stoughton.

Thorne, B. (ed) (1990) 'Symposium: spiritual dimensions in counselling', *British Journal of Guidance & Counselling*, vol 18, no 3.

Von Franz, M.-L. (1986) *On Dreams and Death, a Jungian Interpretation*, Boston, MA, and London: Shamhala.

SUICIDE AND EUTHANASIA

Davies, J. (1997) *Choice in Dying: The Facts about Voluntary Euthanasia*, (foreword by Dirk Bogarde), London: Ward Lock.

The Advance Directive, London: The Voluntary Euthanasia Society.

The Samaritans (1996) *The Cost of Stress*, Slough: The Samaritans.

The Samaritans (1996) *Challenging the Taboo: Attitudes Towards Suicide and Depression*, Slough: The Samaritans.

The Samaritans (1997) *Exploring the Taboo: Attitudes of Young People towards Suicide and Depression*, Slough: The Samaritans.

The Samaritans (1998) *Listen Up: Responding to People in Crisis*, Slough: The Samaritans.

Wertheimer, A. (1991) *A Special Scar: The Experience of People Bereaved by Suicide*, London: Routledge.

PEOPLE AND WORK: BEREAVEMENT, COUNSELLING AND HELPING SKILLS

Adams, A. (1992) *Bullying at Work*, London: Virago.

Bagshaw, M. (2000) *Using Emotional Intelligence at Work*, Ely: Fenman.

Bagshaw, M. (2003) *The Emotionally Intelligent Team*, Ely: Fenman.

Feltham, C. (ed) (1997) *The Gains of Listening: Perspectives on Counselling at Work*, Buckingham: Open University Press.

Graves, D. (2002) *Overcoming Bullying in the Workplace*, London: McGraw Hill.

Mackay, I. (1998) *Listening Skills*, Management Shapers series, London: Institute of Personnel and Development.

Moores, R. (1994) *Managing For High Performance*, London: The Industrial Society (now The Work Foundation).

Murgatoyd, S. and Woolfe, R. (1982) *Coping with Crisis: Understanding and Helping People in Need*, London: Harper & Row.

Reddy, M. (1987) *The Manager's Guide to Counselling at Work*, London: British Psychological Society and Methuen.

Ryan, K.D. and Oestreich, D.K. (1991) *Driving Fear out of the Workplace*, San Francisco, CA: Jossey-Bass.

Stewart, W. (1992) *An A–Z of Counselling Theory and Practice*, London: Chapman & Hall.

The Work Foundation (2002) *Training Pack – Bereavement Issues in the Workplace*, London: The Work Foundation.

Trades Union Congress (1991) *A TUC Charter for Carers*, London: Trades Union Congress.

Trades Union Congress (1994) *A TUC Guide, Family Leave*, London: Trades Union Congress.

Wetton, L. (2003) *A Study into 'The Individual and Organisational Responses to Coping with Bereavement in the Workplace'*, Southampton: Southampton Institute.

Organisations supporting the bereaved

SOME RELEVANT ORGANISATIONS

Some of these and other organisations are listed in the Counselling & Psychotherapy Resources Directory, produced periodically by:

BACP, the British Association for Counselling and Psychotherapy

1 Regent Place, Rugby CV21 2PJ
Telephone 0870 443 5252

Asian Family Counselling Services

Suite 51, The Lodge, 2–4 Windmill Lane, Southall, Middlesex UB2 4NJ
Telephone: 020 8571 3933 Monday to Friday 9 am–4 pm

Counsellors are able to offer caring, personal and confidential counselling in the clients' language with an awareness of their cultural and ethnic backgrounds.

British Humanist Association

1 Gower Street, London WC1E 6HD
Telephone: 020 7079 3580
Email: info@humanism.org.uk

Provides help with non-religious funerals.

Cancerlink

11–21 Northdown Street, London N1 9BN
Telephone: 020 7833 2818
Website: www.cancerlink.org
Freephone cancer information helpline: 0800 132 905 Monday to Friday
    9.30 am–5 pm;
Freephone MAC helpline for young people: 0800 591 028 Monday to
    Friday 9.30 am–5 pm;

Freephone Asian cancer information helpline in Bengali, Hindi, Punjabi, Urdu and English: 0800 590 415 Monday 10 am–1 pm and Friday 10 am–4 pm

Provides emotional support and information to people with cancer, their families, friends and health professionals. Produces a range of publications and acts as a resource for over 600 cancer self-help and support groups throughout the UK via training and development with the latest information on different types of cancer.

CancerBACUP

3 Bath Place, Rivington Street, London EC2A 3JR
Freephone helpline: 0808 800 1234 Monday to Friday 9 am–7 pm

Provides information about cancer or its treatment, with specialist cancer nurses to answer telephone calls, letters or emails about all types and aspects of cancer including: diagnosis, treatment, symptom control, clinical trials, support groups, where to get help and every other facet of coping with cancer.

The Chartered Institute of Personnel and Development (CIPD)

CIPD House, Camp Road, London SW19 4UX
Website: www.cipd.co.uk

Aims to lead in the development and promotion of good practice in the field of the management and development of people.

The Child Bereavement Network

Telephone: 0115 911 8070
Email: cbn@ncb.org.uk

A national resource for bereaved children, young people, their families and other caregivers.

The Child Bereavement Trust

Aston House, West Wycombe, High Wycombe, Bucks HP14 3AG
Telephone: Administration: 01494 446 648 Information and support: 0845 357 1000
Email: enquiries@childbereavement.org.uk
Website: www.childbereavement.org.uk

Launched in 1994, provides support, information and training.

The Compassionate Friends (UK)

53 North Street, Bristol BS3 1EN
Freephone helpline: 08451 232 304 from 10 am–4 pm, 6.30 pm–10.30 pm

An organisation of bereaved parents and their families that offers understanding, support and encouragement to others after the death of a child or
children, including other relatives, friends and professionals who are helping
the family.

Cruse Bereavement Care (UK)

Cruse House, 126 Sheen Road, Richmond, Surrey TW9 1UR
Telephone: Administration: 020 8939 9530 Helpline: 0870 167 1677
Email: helpline@crusebereavementcare.org.uk
Website: www.crusebereavementcare.org.uk

Offers advice, information and support, practical and emotional to all
bereaved people. It is a free service offered by trained supervised volunteers.

The Foundation for the Study of Infant Deaths (FSID)

Artillery House, 11–19 Artillery Row, London SW1P 1RT
Telephone: Administration: 0870 787 0885 Helpline: 0870 787 0554

A counselling service to newly bereaved parents and their families following
the unexpected death of their baby. Cot death is the sudden and unexpected
death of a baby for no obvious reason. The post-mortem examination may
explain some deaths. Those that remain unexplained after post-mortem
examination may be registered as sudden infant death syndrome, SIDS,
sudden infant death, sudden unexpected death in infancy, unascertained or
cot death.

Jewish Bereavement Counselling Service (JBCS)

JBCS, 8/10 Forty Avenue, Wembley HA9 8JW
E-mail: jbcs@jvisit.org.uk

Lesbian and Gay Bereavement Project

Vaughan M Williams Centre, Colindale Hospital, London NW9 5HG
Telephone via Gay switchboard: 0208 455 8894

Telephone support and counselling to those bereaved by the loss of a same-
sex partner.

London Bereavement Network

356 Holloway Road, London N7 6PA
Telephone: 020 7700 8134
email: info@bereavement.org.uk
Website: www.bereavement.org.uk

Bereaved people can contact the group to find the name of a local group for bereavement counselling. Offers support, training and guidelines to all bereavement services in Greater London.

National Association of Bereavement Services

2nd Floor, 4 Pinchin Street, London E1 1SA
Telephone: 020 7709 9090
Helpline: 0171 247 1080 Monday to Friday 10 am–4 pm

A nationwide network of organisations and individuals offering services to bereaved people. Provides information about the nearest, most appropriate source of support.

Office of Fair Trading

Funerals website: www.oft.gov.uk, 'A consumer's guide to funerals'.

RoadPeace (the national charity for road traffic accident victims)

PO Box 2579, London NW10 3PW
Helpline: 0845 4500 355
Email: info@roadpeace.org

Established in 1992 to respond to the need for an organisation supporting those bereaved or injured in a road crash, working for real road safety and representing and supporting this huge group of victims and drawing attention to their almost non-existent rights.

The Samaritans

The Upper Mill, Kingston Road, Ewell, Surrey KT17 2AF
Helpline: 08457 909 090

Provides confidential support 24 hours a day for those who feel suicidal or despairing.

Stillbirth and Neonatal Death Society (SANDS)

28 Portland Place, London W1B 1LY
Telephone: 01189 889 797 (24-hour answerphone)
Email: support@uk-sands.org

Provides help to individuals or couples by way of befriending or group support from parents who have suffered a similar bereavement.

Sudden Death Support Association

Dolphin House, Part Lane, Swallowfield, Reading, Berkshire RG7 1BB
Telephone: 01189 889 797 (24-hour answerphone)

Supports the relatives and close friends of those who die suddenly.

Support After Murder and Manslaughter (SAMM)

Cranmer House, 39 Brixton Road, London SW9 6DZ
Telephone: 020 7735 3838
Email: enquiries@samm.org.uk

Offers emotional support to those bereaved through murder and manslaughter. As part of support for families, attempts to make society more aware of the devastating effects of these dreadful crimes.

Survivors of Bereavement by Suicide (SOBS)

Centre 88, Saner Street, Hull HU3 2TR
Telephone: 01482 610 728 Helpline: 0870 241 3337 Every day 9 am–
    9 pm

Offers emotional and practical support to those bereaved by the suicide of a close relative or friend.

Terence Higgins Trust

52–54 Grays Inn Road, London WC1X 8JU
Telephone: Administration: 020 7831 0330 Helpline: 0845 1221 200
Monday to Friday 10 am – 10 pm, Saturday to Sunday 12 noon–6 pm.
Website: www.tht.org.uk

Provides information, advice and support for those who are concerned that they may be HIV positive or have AIDS.

Trades Union Congress (TUC)

Congress House, Great Russell Street, London WC1B 3LS
Telephone: 020 7636 4030

With 71 affiliated unions representing nearly seven million working people from all walks of life, campaigns for a fair deal at work and for social justice at home and abroad.

Winston's Wish

Telephone: 0845 203 0405
Website: www.winstonswish.org.uk

Founded in 1992 to help bereaved children and young people rebuild their lives after a family death, offers practical support and guidance to families, professionals and anyone concerned about a grieving child.

The Work Foundation

Peter Runge House, 3 Carlton House Terrace, London SW1Y 5DG
Telephone: 0870 165 6700

Provides help, information and advice on people management issues.

Index